CW00505831

ACID
REFLUX DIET

The Ultimate Guide to Enjoying 200 Healthy Recipes and Good Food without Stomach Risks to Manage Heartburn and Acidity. 21-day meal plan to facilitate and improve digestion.

Cheryl Shea

© Copyright 2021 by Cheryl Shea -
All rights reserved.

The following Book is reproduced below with the goal of providing information that is as accurate and reliable as possible. Regardless, purchasing this Book can be seen as consent to the fact that both the publisher and the author of this book are in no way experts on the topics discussed within and that any recommendations or suggestions that are made herein are for entertainment purposes only. Professionals should be consulted as needed prior to undertaking any of the action endorsed herein.

This declaration is deemed fair and valid by both the American Bar Association and the Committee of Publishers Association and is legally binding throughout the United States.

Furthermore, the transmission, duplication, or reproduction of any of the following work including specific information will be considered an illegal act irrespective of if it is done electronically or in print. This extends to creating a secondary or tertiary copy of the work or a recorded copy and is only allowed with the express written consent from the Publisher. All additional right reserved.

The information in the following pages is broadly considered a truthful and accurate account of facts and as such, any inattention, use, or misuse of the information in question by the reader will render any resulting actions solely under their purview. There are no scenarios in which the publisher or the original author of this work can be in any fashion deemed liable for any hardship or damages that may befall them after undertaking information described herein.

Additionally, the information in the following pages is intended only for informational purposes and should thus be thought of as universal. As befitting its nature, it is presented without assurance regarding its prolonged validity or interim quality. Trademarks that are mentioned are done without written consent and can in no way be considered an endorsement from the trademark holder.

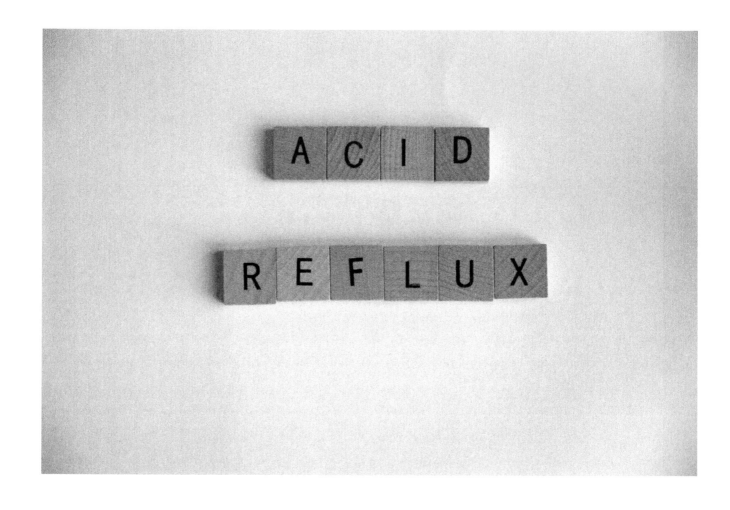

Table of Contents

CAPITOLO 16: SWEETS NOT TO BURDEN THE STOMACH

CONCLUSION

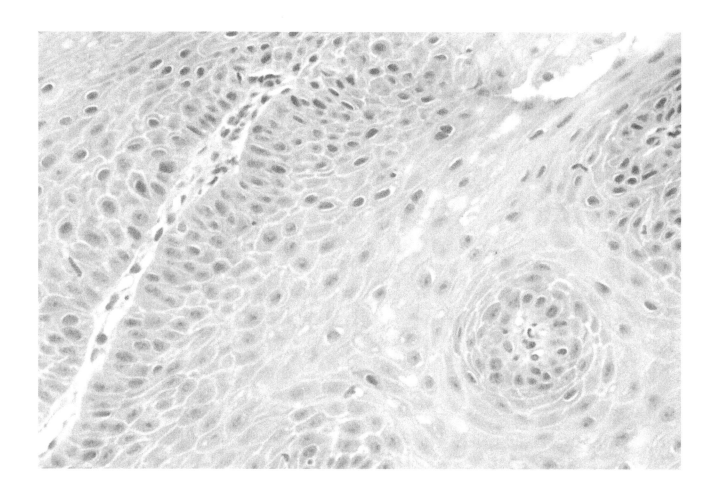

Introduction

What Is Acid Reflux?

When someone suffers from acid reflux, a burning and intense pain in the chest is usually emitted. The person with acid reflux may also suffer from a sour taste and a bitter regurgitation or belching. The acid reflux may be caused by heartburn but may also be related to gastroesophageal reflux disease (GERD). For the most part, GERD occurs when stomach contents are pushed back into the esophagus. But on top of that, it can lead to a hiatal hernia. People who have GERD often need surgery or medication to experience relief. However, a diet may help relieve some symptoms or completely cure the condition. There are many different types of acid reflux that an individual can suffer from. These include Zollinger Strauss Syndrome, which is also known as Zollinger-Ellison syndrome. Hiatal hernia is another form of acid reflux associated with GERD symptoms, such as heartburn. The major difference between GERD and hiatal hernia is that the latter produces pain in the chest. At the same time, GERD causes burning or discomfort in the epigastrium region of the body.

What Is an Acid Reflux Diet?

In the past, one of the easiest ways to treat acid reflux was through diet. Many people will be familiar with the "acid reflux diet," which primarily consists of a low-fat, high-protein diet. The idea is that by avoiding foods high in fat, protein, and simple carbohydrates, one will not cause too much acid to be produced in the stomach, leading to heartburn. As with any diet, it's important to speak to your doctor or health professional before you begin on an acid reflux diet.

Benefits of an Acid Reflux Diet

One of the main benefits of an acid reflux diet is that it improves the stomach's acidity. By doing this, one may avoid heartburn symptoms, such as chest pain. It is also thought to improve digestion by increasing the amount of hydrochloric acid released into the intestines. Other acids, such as pepsin and bile, are also increased, which are thought to aid in digestion. Acid reflux diet is also recommended due to its ability to boost weight loss through "starvation mode." Knowing that it's best to avoid eating after 6 pm due to GERD symptoms, a low-fat, high-protein diet could be used to help lose weight quickly. A low-carb diet that involves avoiding simple carbohydrates, such as sugar, is also good for weight loss—so much of the same applies here. Again, this needs to be done in consultation with a qualified professional. A well-balanced diet is the key to success with acid reflux.

One of the other benefits of an acid reflux diet is that it can positively affect overall health. Studies have shown that those who follow an acid reflux diet also significantly decrease their risk of developing other health complications later in life, such as diabetes, heart disease, and stroke. Acid reflux disease is also known to cause throat cancer; however, going on an acid reflux diet may reduce the risk substantially. It is thought that the nutrients in an acid reflux diet can boost the levels of cancer-fighting compounds, such as lycopene.

An acid reflux diet can also help reduce other negative symptoms. One of these is bloating, which is caused by excess gas. It has been shown that those who go on an acid reflux diet and don't indulge in certain foods, such as beans, onions, carbonated or caffeinated beverages, are less likely to suffer from bloating. Heartburn and indigestion are two other complications that may be reduced with a healthy low-fat, high-protein, and low-carbohydrate diet.

This book contains a complete guide for an acid reflux diet and recipes that will help you maintain your diet in total health.

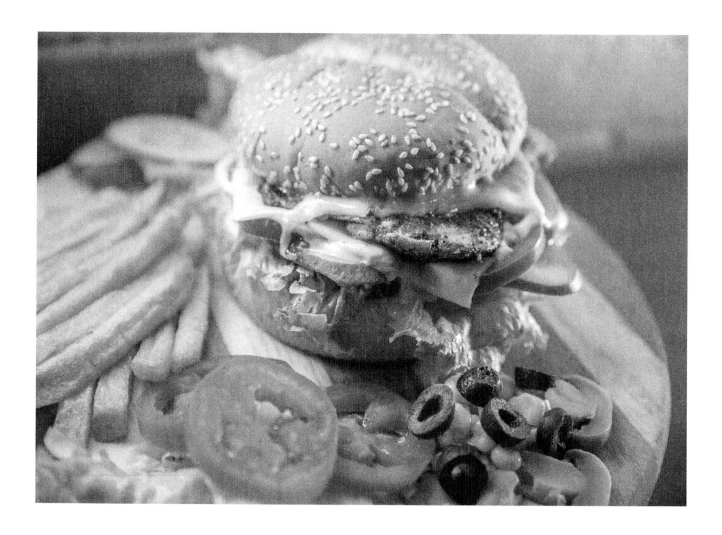

CAPITOLO 1:

Difficult Digestion Because We Find It Hard to Digest

You probably know, or possibly have experienced yourself, that eating certain foods can aggravate indigestion. Perhaps you ate a rich chocolate torte before bedtime and woke up several hours later with a burning in your chest and throat, or maybe a spicy dinner created the need to take antacids a few hours later. Many people have had such experiences and understand that, at least occasionally, eating some foods causes heartburn. There is a strong connection between the foods you eat and acid reflux, GERD, and laryngopharyngeal reflux (LPR). There are three primary ways food can trigger GERD and its variants:

- It can weaken the lower esophageal sphincter (LES).
- It can increase acidity in the stomach.
- It can increase intra-abdominal pressure (IAP).

Acidity and Alkalinity

All substances have the property of pH, which measures the degree of acidity or alkalinity (or neutrality). If you recall basic high school chemistry, the higher the pH of something, the more alkaline it is. The lower the pH, the more acidic it is. A pH of 7 indicates the substance is neutral—that is, neither acidic nor basic. Likewise, you likely learned that adding an alkaline substance to an acidic one neutralizes the acidity. This principle also holds true with food. If you have an ailment linked to high acidity in your stomach, such as acid reflux and its variants, adding acidic foods to that system will make it even more acidic. Adding alkaline foods will help neutralize the acids. Many people seek to neutralize the acids in their stomach with antacids, which are powerful alkaline substances that may neutralize stomach acid. However, the International Foundation for Functional Gastrointestinal Disorders (IFFGD) notes that although these substances are fast-acting, they are also short-term, temporary solutions that may come with their own issues, such as causing rebound acidity (an increase in stomach acidity in response to taking them), as well as other unwanted side effects. However, eating alkaline foods doesn't come with these same risks. Therefore, for permanent relief of acid reflux without side effects, your best bet is to choose alkaline foods and minimize acidic foods.

Food Allergies, Sensitivities, and Intolerances

As I revamped the way I ate, I discovered that one of my biggest acid reflux triggers was related to my food intolerances. What I discovered was that when I consumed food to which I was intolerant, I was far more likely to develop acid reflux than when I did not. That's because food allergies and intolerances affect your body's ability to digest the foods you eat. Consuming them may cause issues that lead to increased IAP because they may…

- delay the emptying of stomach contents.
- cause poor or incomplete digestion.
- cause bloating and gas.
- cause changes in gut bacteria (the gut microbiome).
- cause a condition with symptoms that overlap those of acid reflux.

People may be intolerant, sensitive, or allergic to several common foods or ingredients.

Gluten

According to "BeyondCeliac.org," about 1% of the population has celiac disease—an autoimmune form of gluten intolerance in which sufferers can't process even trace amounts of gluten. However, this number may be higher as experts estimate about 83% of Americans with celiac disease remain undiagnosed or misdiagnosed. The organization further estimates that about 18 million Americans don't have celiac disease, but they still have a gluten intolerance called non-celiac gluten sensitivity. Studies note a strong link between ingestion of gluten in intolerant individuals and acid reflux events. In these individuals with both a gluten intolerance (or celiac disease) and acid reflux, avoiding gluten is incredibly important to manage both conditions.

Dairy Products

For people with intolerance to dairy products (commonly arising from intolerance to the milk sugar lactose or from an allergy to dairy's primary protein casein), GERD is often a co-occurring condition, according to "Healthline." This isn't necessarily because dairy products cause GERD by themselves, but rather because intolerances can cause gas that increases IAP. You must avoid dairy if you are intolerant to it, especially if you are also trying to control acid reflux.

FODMAPS

Some people are sensitive to a certain category of poorly digested carbohydrates called "FODMAPs" (fermentable oligosaccharides, disaccharides, monosaccharides, and polyols). These carbs occur in naturally many foods, ranging from fruit and milk to grains and beans. For people with FODMAP sensitivity, which often manifests as irritable bowel syndrome (IBS), eating these carbohydrates can cause a whole host of gastrointestinal symptoms, including gas, bloating, delayed stomach emptying, and constipation all of which can increase IAP and contribute to GERD. If you've been diagnosed with IBS, or other bowel diseases, like Crohn's disease, inflammatory bowel disease (IBD), or colitis, you may be sensitive to FODMAPs in your diet. For more information about FODMAPs and how to avoid them, visit "Monash University" to learn about the low-FODMAP diet for IBS.

Other Foods

It should also be noted that food allergies can create symptoms that appear to be acid reflux but may actually be a condition called "eosinophilic esophagitis" (EE). According to the Mayo Clinic, EE occurs when white blood cells build up in the esophagus and become symptomatic. While EE occurs due to acid reflux, it has other causes as well, including being a reaction to consuming foods to which one is allergic. The resultant inflammation can cause a host of symptoms similar to GERD (or overlapping with it), such as difficulty swallowing, chest pain that doesn't respond to antacids, persistent heartburn, and regurgitation. If you have GERD symptoms that don't respond (or don't respond as well as you hope) to GERD medications or an acid reflux diet, you may have EE associated with food or substance allergies. Common food allergens that may contribute to EE include the most common allergens—wheat, fish, shellfish, peanuts, tree nuts, dairy, and eggs—and less common allergies to foods. If you suspect food allergies are contributing to your symptoms, talk to your doctor about being tested.

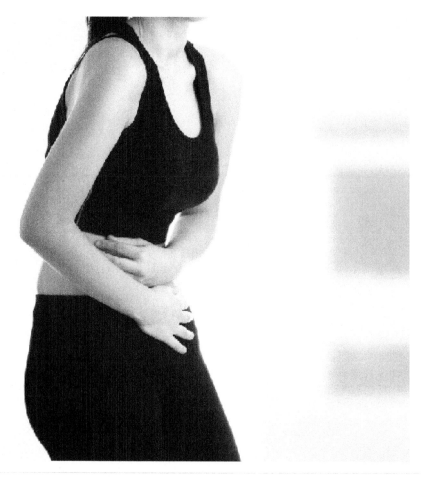

CAPITOLO 2:

Foods that Weigh down the Stomach

Not entirely all foods have the same impact on digestion. However, there are sure foods that have been linked to acid reflux most often. These are typically foods that you may have trouble digesting or ones that alter the amount and acidity of stomach acid as they are being digested. Keep an eye out for these foods in your diet and try to reduce their presence or remove them completely if possible.

Fatty Foods

These foods, particularly those that have been fried, are big offenders of acid reflux. This is because they cause your LES muscle to relax, allowing stomach acid to enter the esophagus. Fatty foods should be avoided by anyone with acid reflux issues since doing so will not only help your LES function properly but also cause you to develop healthier eating habits that can aid in fitness and weight loss.
Even though you will need to steer clear of most fats, your body does need some fat to function. Try to stick to healthier fats, like those found naturally in fish or cooking oils like olive oil and avocado oil when necessary. Use these fats sparingly for best results.

Spicy Foods

Spicy foods are a common cause of acid reflux. Meals that are very hot and spicy typically contain the compound "capsaicin," a naturally occurring source of heat in things like jalapeño peppers, hot sauce, and various spices.
Capsaicin slows your rate of digestion, which gives acid reflux more time to occur as your body processes the meal. Additionally, eating food that is too spicy can irritate your throat, worsening damage and discomfort. Avoid chili peppers, onions, and garlic. Besides, keep black pepper intake to a minimum to reduce acid reflux symptoms.

Acidic Foods

Foods high in acidity can increase the acidity of stomach bile. Any stomach acid that passes through the LES into the esophagus becomes more likely to result in a stronger case of acid reflux. To keep your stomach acid at the correct acidity, cut out low-pH foods from your diet. This includes citrus fruits like lemons, limes, grapefruits, pineapples, and oranges. Tomatoes should also be avoided. Acidity is not just restricted to fruits. Refined grains and sugars are also considered acidic, as are some meat and dairy products.
If you are not looking to go fully vegan or gluten-free, still consider moderating the amount of these foods that you consume and replacing them with alternatives like whole grains and plant-based proteins.

Chocolate and Mint

If you're a big dessert fan, this one may be rough. Chocolate is high in fat, and it also contains tryptophan, a compound that causes your brain to produce serotonin. While this can moderately improve your mood to a certain extent, both serotonin and fat loosen the LES muscle and allow acid reflux to occur. Mint similarly relaxes the LES. Skip the pain and avoid these after-dinner desserts.

Drinks

Water is always your best bet for acid reflux and getting a drink in general, but there are some drinks you should absolutely avoid. Any products high in caffeine are known to cause acid reflux as they stimulate acid production in the stomach. Coffee and tea are both acidic and can cause acid reflux symptoms to worsen, as can acidic fruit juices or those with added sugar. Soda should be avoided, both for the carbonation, which can worsen digestive issues, and the sugar. Consuming too much alcohol can also increase acid reflux. Plain water, coconut water, low-acid smoothies and juices, and plant-based milk (like almond and soy milk) are all safer drink options.

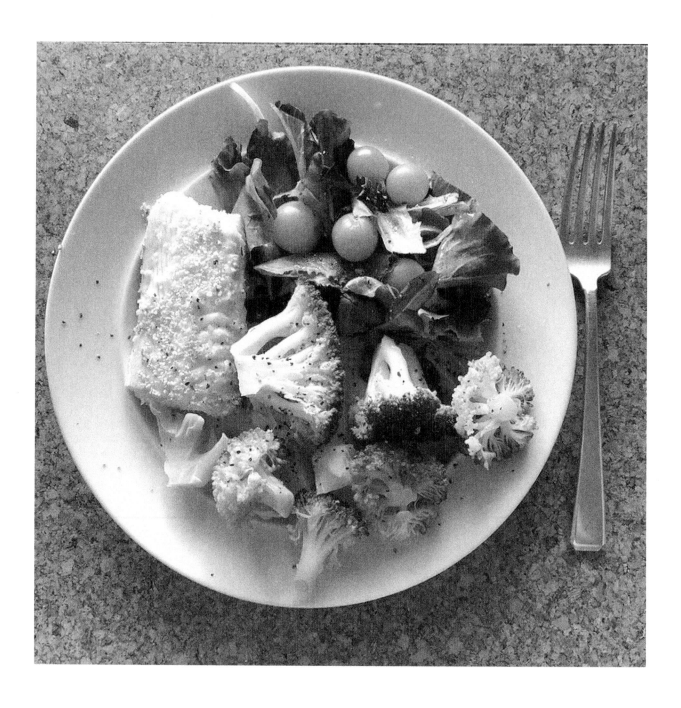

CAPITOLO 3:

Foods that Help Digest Better

The digestive process starts the moment you eat something. The saliva in your mouth breaks down food into smaller molecules like sugars, proteins, and fiber. These break down even further to eventually become nutrients needed by your body. As you swallow these nutrients down the esophagus, they're mixed with stomach acid and enzymes to liquefy them into a thinner liquid called "chyme." This liquid moves through the small intestine, where most of its nutrients are absorbed before being stored in the large intestine for elimination from the body as wastewater or feces.

Some foods provide helpful stimulation for digestion, and here is a small list of foods that help us to digest better:

Oatmeal

It helps in controlling the digestive system, and it can cure diarrhea by making a paste from oatmeal powder mixed with milk and applying this mixture over your stomach.

Water

It is good for overall health and is vital to help in softening stools and prevent constipation. Drinking chilled water or water at room temperature has the same effect as warm water.

Tomatoes

Tomatoes provide two types of fiber that increase bowel movements, which are insoluble fiber (cellulose) and soluble fiber (pectin). Soluble fiber absorbs liquid as it moves through the intestinal tract, which assists in softening stools, thus relieving constipation.

Yogurt

It contains good bacteria that manufacture enzymes, which digest food. A study was conducted at the University of Wisconsin (Madison) where people who consumed the highest amount of yogurt had a significantly greater number and volume of bowel movements.

Wheat Germ

Wheat germ supplements contain increased amounts of B vitamins and vitamin E, which are necessary for the growth and development of healthy bacteria in your body's intestinal tract. This aids in digestion and may help to prevent colon cancer due to its high content of fiber, antioxidants, vitamin E, and other nutrients required for good health.

Bananas

Bananas are a great source of fiber, which is essential for normal bowel movements. The carbohydrate and mineral content of bananas helps in producing good bowel movements. Due to their high content of vitamin A and C, bananas are also excellent for your hands, nails, and hair.

Watermelon Seeds

Watermelon seeds contain high amounts of fiber, antioxidants, manganese, potassium, magnesium, and iron. This makes it an excellent digestive cleanser that can cure constipation, as it's high in fiber.

Papaya Seeds

Papaya seeds contain the proteolytic enzyme papain, which aids in digestion as well as in relieving flatulence (gas). It is also high in vitamin B6 and niacin. It is one of the richest sources of provitamin A.

Broccoli

Broccoli contains a compound called "sulforaphane," which is known to be useful in eradicating harmful bacteria. Broccoli also aids digestion and may relieve gas, bloating, and indigestion, as it contains fiber.

Chia Seeds

Chia seeds contain mucilage, which absorbs water from the digestive system and then releases it to help soften stools and lubricate the intestinal tract. This also helps in reducing cholesterol while simultaneously preventing colon cancer, which is abundant in the bowel.

Garlic

Researchers have found that eating seven cloves each day is enough to cure most cases of halitosis (bad breath) due to a compound called "allicin."

Nightshade Vegetables

Potatoes, tomatoes, eggplants, peppers and solanum. These foods contain the alkaloids "solanine" and "psoralens," which are cytotoxic with potential cancer-releasing properties. Therefore, it is best avoided.

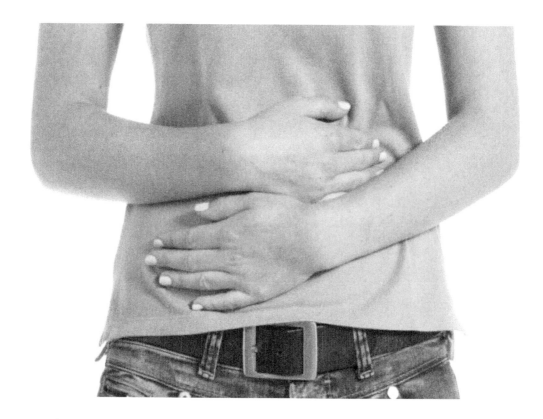

CAPITOLO 4:

Gastritis (The Fire Inside)

Our stomach is protected by a layer of gastric mucosal protection that is carried out on the functions of prostaglandins. These prostaglandins play a key role in protecting the stomach lining from being burned by its own acid. Over time, gastritis occurs as these prostaglandins are gradually decreased by:

- Excessive alcohol intake
- Bacterial infections (such as H. pylori or "helicobacter pylori")
- Certain medications or steroids
- Stressful events, stress from the workplace, and stress from relationships
- Excessive and prolonged anger
- A weak immune system or autoimmunity
- Acid reflux disease
- Prolonged hostile behavior

By definition, gastritis is a common form of stomach upset that causes inflammation or erosion of the stomach walls. In some cases of gastritis, the lining of the stomach may become irritated or infected, and in other cases, the lining of the stomach may become red or swollen, and in severe cases, the inflammation may also lead to bleeding of the stomach lining.

Understanding the Types of Gastritis

The type of gastritis is determined by the condition and causes of the inflammation. Consequently, gastritis may be either acute or chronic, depending on certain factors and the severity of the inflammation.

Acute gastritis inflammation is a very serious condition and is often caused by food poisoning, eating spoiled food, or merely overeating. In this case, the lining of the stomach may also become seriously inflamed following the swallowing of irritating substances, such as poison, lye, or acid. For cases of acute gastritis, two major complications may occur, which are known as gastric obstruction and pernicious anemia. Gastric obstruction, or what is also known as a "gastric outlet obstruction," is a deep tissue inflammation that extends into the muscle lining of the stomach, which causes further inflammation in the gastric outlet. This obstruction prevents food from normally leaving the stomach and may result in vomiting and loss of potassium electrolytes, fluids, and acids. On the other hand, pernicious anemia may occur if there is anything that causes burning of the gastric parietal cells, which are the little cells that line the stomach.

The common symptoms of acute gastritis include:

- Loss of appetite
- A feeling of pressure and fullness in the pit of the stomach (which isn't relieved by belching)
- Nausea
- Vomiting
- Headache
- Heartburn
- Fever
- Fatigue
- An overall sense of sickness

In order to treat acute gastritis, immediate medical attention is needed, and this requires quick actions by a physician to remove the irritating substance. Following the removal of the substance, the treatment may include neutralization of the irritating substance to avoid the stomach wall from becoming perforated and developing acute peritonitis. In some cases of acute gastritis, surgical treatment may also be necessary. Overall, relief from acute gastritis is usually brought about within a few days following the elimination of the irritating substance.

Chronic gastritis inflammation is generally due to some development of an ulcer in the stomach. As mentioned earlier, there are many different conditions that may produce repeated stomach irritations, and the treatment period may span over a long period of time. With this condition, there is often the feeling of fullness soon after eating just small bites of food. In comparison to acute gastritis, which may occur abruptly, chronic gastritis occurs at a much slower pace. Chronic gastritis is treated mainly by counteracting the high amounts of acid that are present in the stomach. By neutralizing the acidity levels in the stomach, it will help in avoiding further stomach lining erosion.

Severe Cases of Gastritis

There may be times when certain symptoms of gastritis are considered to be an emergency situation, which requires immediate medical attention. Here are some serious gastritis symptoms that are considered to require immediate medical attention:

- Swelling in abdomen
- Stomach pain getting worse or moving to lower right abdomen (the appendix area)
- Frequent vomiting (not being able to keep down any food or liquids)
- Frequent diarrhea
- Feelings of dizziness
- Red blood in stool
- Fainting
- Difficulty breathing
- Pain that spreads to the chest, back, arm, neck, or shoulders
- Vomiting blood (red or black)
- Condition keeping deteriorating

CAPITOLO 5:

Foods that Extinguish the Burn

Acid reflux happens once stomach acid comes back up in the esophagus, which is your food pipe. The acid damages the lining of these organs and may irritate your throat, causing heartburns or sour burps.
One of the most common causes of acid reflux is food intake. Acidic foods like citrus fruits and tomatoes can trigger this condition since they promote laxity in these muscles to allow passage for digestion and absorption into the bloodstream, according to a study from Cornell University's On-Line Journal of Biological Sciences.
Some foods help to extinguish the burn that you might be experiencing because of acid reflux, and these are as follows:

Beans
Beans are great for those who suffer from acid reflux as they ensure the proper mixing of bile acids and acids within the body to prevent stomach inflammation. However, it is significant to note that beans are also rich in calories or carbohydrates, so when you resort to them for your diet, be sure to consume low-calorie meal alternatives in addition to them.

Whole Grains
The dietary fiber found in grains and whole-grain foods is good for preventing acid reflux because it keeps food moving over the digestive system without causing digestive tract discomfort. Just make sure that you're including enough fiber-rich foods regularly so that your body can properly absorb its nutrients.

Red Meats
Red meat is rich in protein, which helps to stimulate the production of hydrochloric acid in your stomach. In this way, it contributes to correct digestive system function. However, some red meats contain fat and cholesterol, and these need to be paid attention to, as they may cause damage to your esophagus from increasing acidity levels.

Fish
Fish comprises omega-3 fatty acids, which aid to keep the stomach from becoming inflamed. In some cases, these acids can cause excess acidity within the stomach and esophagus. It is also important that you're including enough healthy fats in your diet as they are needed for the proper functioning of your body and brain.

Spinach
The fiber found in spinach can help in reducing stomach acidity levels by ensuring that foods move through your system smoothly while also providing nutrients that are needed for the proper functioning of your digestive system.

Dark Chocolate
Dark chocolate is rich in magnesium, which will help you address and prevent stomach acid reflux by helping to regulate the muscles that push food through your digestive system. This may also help you to manage a heartburn condition, as it helps in decreasing the levels of stomach acid.

Ginger
Ginger is rich in anti-inflammatory properties that trigger the release of bile acids, which are natural enzymes produced within the liver and pancreas that help balance and control the amount of gastric acid produced within the body.

Protein

Protein is a must, as it helps to prevent acid reflux by its ability to promote digestion and absorption of nutrients. It is also essential for the production and release of hydrochloric acid in your stomach.

Yogurt

Yogurt is great for acid reflux because it can stimulate digestion, which means that foods will be more easily broken down into smaller particles, and chemicals such as bile will be more easily dispersed throughout the body. Yogurt may also contain probiotics that help the body fight off stomach infections that can be caused by too much stomach acid production.

CAPITOLO 6:

Tips to Follow at the Table

For many people, the term "acid reflux" means nothing. But for those who suffer from this painful condition, it is a debilitating disease that makes eating a social nightmare. Acid reflux is instigated by stomach acid dripping upwards into the esophagus. This can be triggered when poor posture or overeating causes excessive pressure on the stomach, as well as when you lie down quickly after eating, which results in gravity pulling food back up towards your throat and increases the production of stomach acids. Consequently, what can you do to halt this? Here are some key tips to remember at the table:

Sit with Your Spine Straight Throughout Your Meal (No Slouching)

It is important to sit straight throughout your meal and avoid slouching at the table. As soon as you slouch, you put an additional burden on your stomach, which can lead to more heartburn or indigestion. So, try to avoid laying down immediately after eating, and keep your head level with the rest of your body throughout the meal. This will help you stop stomach acid from building up in your stomach and enter your esophagus, where it causes severe pain and discomfort.

Eat Slowly

While eating slowly helps reduce the impact of overeating, it is essential to avoid eating so quickly that you do not fully chew or swallow. You may think that you are eating slowly, but the truth is, you may be eating so quickly that you are not even taking the time to chew and swallow. This can cause indigestion and lead to excessive stomach acid built up in your stomach, which causes pain and discomfort in your esophagus.

Chew Well

According to a study, people who do not chew well during a meal suffer higher rates of acid reflux. When you do not chew well, your food gets stuck in the back of your throat, which can cause severe irritation and pain as stomach acid builds up.

Eat at Least Three Hours Before Bedtime

Eating close to bedtime or before sleeping has been shown to impact your ability to fall asleep and reduce the quality of sleep. When you eat too close to bedtime, your body tends to spend more energy digesting food rather than relaxing; this can lead to poor sleep quality and stressful dreams. So, make sure that you avoid eating at least three hours before going to bed. This will help ensure that you get a good night's rest and wake up refreshed in the morning.

Avoid Alcohol

Alcohol can make acid reflux worse, according to several studies, and it is known to increase the production of stomach acids. So, avoid drinking alcohol during an acidic meal. But if you do drink alcohol, it is best to limit the amount you drink and be cautious about when you drink it since there are negative side effects that can occur following heavy drinking.

Avoid Tuna Fish and Shark in Packing

Avoid eating tuna fish two hours before bedtime as this can lead to heartburn since tuna fish contains a lot of mercury, which impacts the way your body processes food, leaving more sodium in the stomach than your body needs. However, it is okay to eat tuna fish two hours before bedtime. So, avoid these foods completely when you are about to go to bed.

Avoid Dairy Products Before Bedtime

Reduced levels of dairy products in the body can lead to acid reflux and indigestion, which also increase your risk of reflux disease, GERD, or heartburn. It is best to avoid dairy products when going to bed, as they can upset your stomach and cause acid reflux. But it is okay for a small number of dairy products such as yogurt, cottage cheese, or melon every day throughout the day if you want them so that you get a minimal amount of the bacteria that could potentially make you sick.

CAPITOLO 7:

Reflux and How to Stop the Fire Rising from the Stomach

Gastric acid reflux is not a chronic disease, and people usually feel reflux after having a certain food. It is normal in several cases, and it can be eliminated or reduced with certain medical or natural remedies. But if it is not treated well, or a person is having some digestive system problem, the problem can be persistent and become worse. The chronic disease of acid reflux refers to gastroesophageal reflux diseases. It usually occurs when a person constantly feels acid or food between the canal tube that is linked between the stomach and throat. It is also known as "heartburn" and creates discomfort and other potential risks to a person's health. In this scenario, a person feels or experiences the undigested food or stomach content in the food tube and in the throat. It can damage the inner lining of the tube and the stomach walls as well.

Acid reflux quickly influences people who have any other health complications. For example, it is common in those with both type 1 and type 2 diabetes. People with asthma may also suffer from acid reflux. Poor digestion problems or other stomach-related diseases can also create acid reflux. The treatment of this problem is necessary to be done on time to overcome other health complications, and if not done, then this can cause multiple serious consequences.

According to research, it is shown that acid reflux can be due to improper food intake and consumption of too much fried food and carbonated drinks. This can weaken the power of the stomach to digest the food easily, and it can become reactive towards it. Sometimes other health problems can be behind gastric acid reflux. But during the initial stages, with the little concentration of food intake and lifestyle changes, the problem can easily be treated and overcome before it becomes a significant problem.

Treatment of Acid Reflux

Due to poor lifestyles and unhealthy routines, this leads to different health problems, and acid reflux is one of them. Our lives are too much occupied, and it is hard to find "time" to eat at the "right time." This increases bad food choices and leads to inappropriate meal times. This increases the weight of a person and can lead to obesity. These activities directly impact your sleep and mind activity. When a person does not have a sound mind and feels restless, the digestive system is the most sensitive part of the whole body. This system feels the effects of the stress first. This leads to inappropriate food digestion and increases acid reflux.

According to doctors and health advisors, acid reflux is a treatable problem, and with some lifestyle changes, it can be overcome easily. In the treatment of acid reflux, the first thing that matters is diagnosis. In the first recommendation, foods that are not allowed to consume include fried and fatty food items, processed and canned food, carbonated drinks, alcoholic drinks, citrus, and pepper. These foods can increase heartburn and a restless condition and can create irritation or damage. Other than the food restriction, it is necessary to reduce the size of the meal that a person consumes in a day. A large meal size can fill the stomach and increase the reaction or irritation. But with smaller meal sizes, the stomach can have a large space, and as a result, this reduces the refluxes. As well as it is necessary to take the last meal 3 hours before going to sleep, so do not consume food right before bedtime.

To neutralize the condition, keep your head parallel to the body when you are on the bed. It helps in controlling the flow of food or acid towards the food canal and relieves heartburn at nighttime. Do not use a high pillow because it puts exertion or pressure on the stomach and can create a restless condition.

With the lifestyle and dietary changes implemented, keep consulting the doctor and get medication as well. The medication can help you neutralize the reflux impact or prevent the acid reflux from gaining a serious impact on your health.

Complications Due to Acid Reflux

Acid reflux is a digestive-related problem that can be treated with medication and a lifestyle change. But if not treated properly, and if the condition is allowed to go untreated for a long time, then it can affect the stomach and other body parts as well. It is reflux or backflow of stomach acid or food towards the food canal that creates heartburn. Due to the movement of the fluid in the throat, a person may experience irritation and dry cough as well. A person with gastric acid reflux usually feels pain in the chest that feels like heart pain, but it is actually due to the gas and the effect of reflux that comes from the stomach. Sometimes the symptoms get worse if not treated on time. Acid reflux can damage the inner lining of the esophagus or can be a reason for bleeding as well. This complication can create a stomach ulcer or can be chronic with time. Due to untreated stomach acid reflux, it is also noticed that some people even face the chronic problem of narrowing of their esophagus lining. With time, it can be the cause of esophageal cancer as well. This severe complication cannot just affect the person's health but also can be the cause of limited activities or reduced productivity. In the worst scenario, these can be life-threatening as well. The best remedy to avoid such issues is to keep the focus on a small problem and get the proper treatment from the health advisor on time.

If you are at the initial stage or facing acid reflux, then it is important to pay attention to your activities. With just small changes in their diet and lifestyle, a person cannot just overcome the issue but also get the treatment they need on time. Even with the natural food and home-based remedies, it is easy to treat and control acid reflux. All you need is to avoid the unhealthy or acidic food choices that increase the acidity in the stomach. Consume the food with minimum spices and salt, which reduces the irritation. Also, have small meal sizes throughout the day. Furthermore, we have some recipes that will help you make delicious meals that offer relief for acid reflux as well.

CAPITOLO 8:

Typical Symptoms

People experience the classic symptoms of heartburn soon after eating. Large meals that are greasy, starchy, or spicy are more problematic. Symptoms are worse if you eat too quickly, lie down, or exercise soon after eating. With silent reflux (LPR), the symptoms can be chronic or intermittent. They may happen around meals or away from meals, during the day or at night.

These are the most common symptoms of reflux, GERD, and LPR:

- Heartburn
- Regurgitation
- Chest pain
- Shortness of breath
- Hoarseness
- Difficulty swallowing
- "Lump" feeling in the throat
- Choking sensation
- Chronic cough
- Chronic throat clearing
- Postnasal drip
- Difficulty breathing
- Intermittent airway obstruction
- Wheezing

The reflux symptom index (RSI) below is a screening tool developed by Drs. Jamie Koufman and Jordan Stern that can help you determine if you have LPR. It doesn't replace a complete medical assessment and diagnosis, but it allows you to see how many related symptoms you have and how severe they are. A score of 15 or higher is an indicator of LPR, but even if you have a lower value and suspect that you have it, it's not a bad idea to check with an ENT specialist.

Within the last month, how did the following problem affect you? (0–5 rating scale, where 0 = no problem and 5 = severe problem)

Hoarseness or problem with your voice	0	1	2	3	4	5
Clearing your throat	0	1	2	3	4	5
Excess throat mucus or postnasal drip	0	1	2	3	4	5
Difficulty swallowing foods, liquids, or pills	0	1	2	3	4	5
Cough after you ate or after lying down	0	1	2	3	4	5
Breathing difficulties or choking episodes	0	1	2	3	4	5
Troublesome or annoying cough	0	1	2	3	4	5
A sensation of something sticking in your throat	0	1	2	3	4	5
Heartburn, chest pain, indigestion, or stomach acid coming up	0	1	2	3	4	5
Total						

Emergency Tips to Treat Flare-ups

If you have heartburn flare-up, you can try one of these remedies:

- **Ginger:** To boost digestion, make a ginger tea by mixing 1 teaspoon of grated fresh ginger in 1 cup of warm water. You may add ½ teaspoon of pure maple syrup if desired.
- **"Aloe vera" Plant:** You may have seen Aloe vera drinks in stores, but these tend to contain sugars and preservatives. Instead, keep an aloe leaf in your refrigerator or grow a plant in your home. Cut a piece of aloe and peel the hard green skin, and you'll be left with the clear, gooey part. Mix it into a smoothie.
- **Bone Broth:** Sipping warm bone broth can help soothe the lining of your throat and esophagus.
- **Get up:** Or, if you're lying down, elevate your head with pillows, so your head is higher than your torso.
- **Rest:** If you're running around catching up on work or errands, stop and take a moment to calm down. Sit down for five minutes and take deep breaths.
- **Walk It off:** If you overate, go out for a light walk. Avoid jumping or any exercise that involves too much shaking.

When Should I See a Doctor?

If you've tried my eating plans and modified your diet for two to four weeks and still continue to experience symptoms, you may want to see a gastroenterologist or ENT (otolaryngologists) doctor. They'll be able to screen you for various disorders ranging from Barrett's esophagus to ulcers and cancer. If there's a serious condition, the sooner you discover it, the better your chances of making a full recovery.

If you have at the least one of these indications, you may want to schedule an appointment with a specialist sooner rather than later:

- Severe heartburn that happens more than twice a week despite following the plans in this book and/or taking over-the-counter acid-suppressing medications for more than two weeks
- Severe chest pain right after eating that almost feels like a heart attack (this usually calls for a trip to your gastroenterologist, but of course chest pain may also mean a heart attack; if it's accompanied by other heart attack signs, such as pain and tightness in the neck and arms, light-headedness, abnormal heartbeat, or anxiety, call 911 right away)
- Extreme coughing that wakes you up at night (especially if it's so severe that you feel you will suffocate or run out of breath)
- A cough that lasts more than three months despite normal chest X-rays and ruling out any chest or throat infections
- Pain or difficulty when swallowing, a choking sensation, or a constant feeling of a lump in the throat
- Hoarseness in the morning that gets worse during the day, or a scratchy voice
- A feeling of narrowing or obstruction in the esophagus
- Nausea or vomiting (especially if vomiting blood, as it can be a sign of esophageal ulcer)
- Blood in the stool or black bowel movements

To help your doctor make a diagnosis, keep a record of your symptoms, the times they happen, and their severity. Record when, what, and how much you eat. Tracking your stress level and sleep will reveal how your environment affects your symptoms. Your symptoms will likely improve, but if they don't, your doctor will want to know that.

Medical tests and doctors' visits may seem unpleasant or stressful. However, ruling out more serious medical conditions will alleviate anxiety and allow you to focus on preparing and eating the right foods. And if the tests do come back with bad news, you'll be able to start treatment sooner and have a better outcome.

CAPITOLO 9:

The Main Causes

There is not one single cause of acid reflux, but it could be one or a combination of many factors causing the problem. It is a doctor's job to help the patient identify these possible causes to create a treatment plan. We will study several potential causes before jumping to any conclusions.

The simplest, widely accepted cause of acid reflux is the production of too much acid in the stomach. As food enters the stomach, it triggers the release of stomach acid into the mix to begin breaking down the food into smaller particles. The amount that is released is usually dependent on how much food and what type of food needs to be broken down. For example, low-fiber foods and simple sugars (like refined flour products) are quickly broken down into their smallest form and therefore do not require much stomach acid to digest. More complex particles, like animal proteins or high-fiber foods, will need a bit more acid to break them down.

If this recognition system gets out of whack, food may trigger a release of stomach acid that is not appropriate for the food. When an overwhelming amount of acid quickly dissolves the food, it is released from the stomach into the small intestine. If the stomach is still producing acid on an empty stomach, it is likely to cause a problem. In the case where too much acid is produced, reflux symptoms are more likely to occur.

The pharmaceutical industry thrives on this concept, as there are several prescriptions and over-the-counter remedies that work by reducing stomach acid. The theory is that if there were less stomach acid altogether, there would be less that would enter the esophagus, therefore relieving symptoms and causing less damage.

Functional Issues Leading to GERD

There are also many functional problems in the esophagus and stomach region that can lead to acid reflux. When food enters the mouth and slides down the esophagus toward the stomach, the lower esophageal sphincter (LES) opens to let the bolus (chewed mass of food) into the stomach, then it closes quickly behind the bolus, protecting the esophagus from any acid that tries to enter. The LES is finely tuned to open at the specific moment the bolus reaches it. If there is any confusion in this signaling, or if there were nerve damage, for example, the LES may begin to open at inappropriate times, allowing stomach acid to enter the esophagus.

The lower esophageal sphincter can also become distorted or twisted, which does not allow it to close completely. This can either be a structural issue or stomach issues. When there is increased pressure in the stomach, it pushes up on the lower esophageal sphincter, opening it slightly. When the seal of the sphincter is compromised, any bit of acid that splashes up through it will cause burning and a painful sensation usually called heartburn. Excess food in the stomach can cause pressure, usually by eating too fast. There may also be a functional issue with the stomach, which causes it to empty slower, allowing food to build up, causing the pressure.

A hiatal hernia is another possible cause of consistent reflux. A hiatal hernia occurs when you get a larger than normal opening in the diaphragm where the esophagus pokes through to meet the stomach. This extra space allows a portion of the stomach to protrude through, causing extra pressure on the lower esophageal sphincter. There is a high possibility of acid entering the esophagus.

A hiatal hernia can happen at birth or develop over time, and it can range in size, leading to different symptoms. Most hernias are harmless and go unnoticed unless a doctor suspects it is the cause of symptoms. Diet changes can address most of the cases, but surgery can fix more severe cases.

Stress and Acid Reflux

Stress seems to be a common culprit in many body ailments. It can cause headaches that turn to migraines, create fatigue, muscle aches, high blood pressure, and several other problems, including acid reflux and GERD. According to a 2011 study reported on "Healthline," there is a strong correlation between work-induced stress and the incidence of GERD. Participants reported a higher rate of GERD during times of stress. This study was completed in Norway with over 40,000 people. They also reported that low job satisfaction was a common thread.

Another study in 1993 shows that more anxious people reported a higher severity of symptoms than people who were generally relaxed. Interestingly, the study established no correlation between these increased feelings of discomfort and a tangible increase in stomach acid. This leads to the theory that stress must have some effect on receptors in the cells of tissue that makes them more sensitive to stimuli, creating the illusion of more symptoms. The doctors theorize that stress somehow turns up sensory receptors in the brain, causing more of a reaction than would normally be induced by a small amount of acid in the esophagus. It proves that symptoms can appear to be exaggerated during stressful times.

Note that the patients involved in this study already reported having symptoms of acid reflux and this was a study to determine the role of stress and increasing signs of GERD. It does not propose that stress causes acid reflux necessarily, just that symptoms can appear worse if stress is a factor.

Also, these studies are limited in that they have only studied the result of acute stress on acid reflux, like exposure to freezing temperatures or loud, annoying noises in controlled environments. They did not test chronic, consistent stress sometimes caused by strained living situations, financial problems, illness, or long-term problems at work. While acute stresses do exist, the majority of people suffer from long-term, deep-seated stressors over time.

While none of the earlier studies found an increase in stomach acid as a result of stress, one interesting study from 1990 found a correlation with stress-induced increases in stomach acid. It found that people with certain personality traits respond differently to stress, and this response either increases or decreases the production of stomach acid. They found that people who are generally laid back and analytical tend to have decreased stomach acid when exposed to acute stressors. On the contrary, people who are more emotional and quicker to react have elevated stomach acid when stress is introduced. This shows again that there is something more going on with stress and acid reflux, yet the causality is still unclear.

To consider another side of the story, we also know that breathing changes as a result of stress. While a calm, resting person will take long, deep breaths, a person under stress will begin to take shallow, short breaths. The response is as old as the human race. In times of acute stress, labeled the "fight or flight" response, early humans would need to increase the oxygen entering the body to prepare for a possible "fight or flight" situation. In response to the stress of possible harm or death, the heart rate quickens, and breathing quickens to supply more oxygen to muscles, including the heart. This is an involuntary body function, so there is no control over it unless you are aware it is occurring and you consciously try to control your breathing. The unfortunate side effect of shallow breathing is a decrease in strength in the muscles that surround the lower esophageal sphincter. Deep breathing allows these muscles to stretch to their maximum and then contract. Shallow breathing uses only a small amount of muscle capacity to work. It would be like doing a bicep curl at the gym and only flexing the muscle halfway. The whole muscle is not being worked out; therefore, it weakens over time.

This is an excellent theory to help explain why stress leads to acid reflux. When chronic stress is present, the likelihood of shallow breathing increases. The muscles around the lower esophageal sphincter weaken, leaving the lower esophageal sphincter unsupported and ready to let in unwanted stomach acid.

Bacteria and GERD

Emerging science is beginning to pinpoint the microbiome, a collection of multiple beneficial bacterial strains living in the gut, as a cause of pressure. It is well known that a variety of bacteria called the "gastrointestinal system home" usually provide several services to the body in exchange for space to live. Bacteria aid in the breakdown and absorption of vitamins and minerals and help in regulating the digestive process. Good, non-harmful strains of bacteria in large colonies help in keeping smaller colonies of harmful bacteria in check. They act as an extension to the immune system. This is why yogurt is recommended to help with digestive issues. The bacteria present in cultured yogurt helps in increasing the colonies of good bacteria living in the gut, therefore aiding in the digestive process and maintaining the populations of harmful bugs.

Bacteria feed on several nutrients, but the most popular are simple sugars broken down from carbohydrate-rich foods, such as pasta, bread, and fruit. As the bacteria feed on these nutrients, they create gas as a byproduct. The simpler the sugars to feed on, the more gas the colony will produce. The gases have nowhere to go but up, settling in the stomach and building pressure. When the lower esophageal sphincter opens to relieve some pressure, it lets the opportunistic stomach acid in, reaching and damaging the esophageal lining. While beneficial bacteria help the body break down food, harmful strains, like Helicobacter pylori (H. pylori for short), cause more stomach acid to be produced, thus exacerbating acid reflux symptoms. The human body has a long history of exposure to H. pylori and therefore knows how to rid itself of it. H. Pylori is sensitive to stomach acid and thrives in a neutral or alkaline environment. The body increases the release of stomach acid in response to the presence of the bacteria. H. pylori is a tough bug to get rid of, so the stomach acid is raised typically for longer periods, resulting in consistent reflux symptoms. As the stomach cells are exposed to more acid than normal for a long period, peptic ulcers begin to develop. If left untreated, the ulcers bleed, leaking much-needed blood from the body. If persistent, nutrient deficiencies and other significant problems develop through the loss of blood. Not to mention, the condition is very painful. Shooting, stabbing pain is a common complaint. Along with stomach acid-reducing agents, a patient is likely to need antibiotics to help the body fight against H. pylori infection.

Pregnancy

Acid reflux can be observed in women during their first pregnancy due to the increased pressure from the gradually growing fetus in addition to enhanced levels of hormones. It is at its peak in the third trimester, and the symptoms of acid reflux start fading away soon after delivery.

Smoking

Apart from increasing the danger of esophagus cancer, the following harmful effects of smoking are considered to be responsible for causing acid reflux:

- Enhancement of acid secretion
- Reduced muscle function of LES
- Reduced production of saliva (saliva is effective in acid neutralization)
- Damaged mucus membranes
- Impaired reflexes of throat muscles

Diet

Lying in bed immediately after consuming food or having a larger meal can result in initiating heartburn and various other symptoms of acid reflux, i.e., problems in food swallowing, dry cough, etc.

The following everyday foods are known to cause acid reflux:

- Carbonated drinks
- Alcohol
- Spicy foods, e.g., chilies and curries
- Chocolate
- Tea (with tea leaves) or coffee (including both decaffeinated and regular)
- Citrus fruits, i.e., lemons, oranges, etc.
- Fried or fatty foods
- Onion and garlic
- Food containing tomato, e.g., pizza, salsa, and spaghetti sauce
- There are many other reasons for acid reflux including:
- Obesity and overweight
- Eating right before sleeping
- Consuming larger meals and afterward either bending over at the waist or lying in bed
- Consuming muscle relaxants, various BP-controlling medications (blood pressure), and even aspirin or ibuprofen, etc.

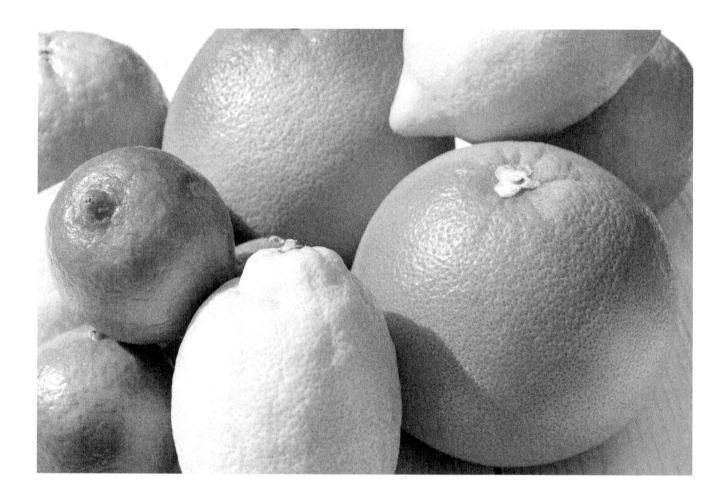

CAPITOLO 10:

Foods to Be Preferred

What to Eat

The below foods will help you manage the symptoms of acid reflux. When you feel the acid reflux coming on, try and eat one or more of these foods to help yourself. Don't get discouraged if you eat something and don't feel a huge difference. Eventually, you will find the foods that work the best for you.

Vegetables

We all know that vegetables are good for us. If anything, adding more vegetables to your diet will increase the amount of nutrients your body is getting. They are naturally low in fat and acid. Some good options are leafy green vegetables, potatoes, cucumber, broccoli, and cauliflower.

Ginger

Please don't think that you have to chomp down on a whole thumb of ginger. Thankfully, you do not need a lot of it to gain the benefits. A great way to incorporate ginger into your diet is to add sliced or crushed pieces to your food or smoothies. You could also make ginger tea. Ginger is a natural anti-inflammatory food and is very good for many gastrointestinal problems.

Oats

Anything high in fiber is beneficial for your digestive system and can help relieve acid reflux. Oats are easy to make and have a lot of fiber in them. You can easily incorporate it into your diet by having it for breakfast with fruit.

Non-Citruscitrus Fruit

Fruit is generally very good for you, so you will do your body good if you increase the amount you eat. Citrus is high in acid, and that is why you should be avoiding those types of fruit. Some of the fruit that you can incorporate into your diet are bananas, apples, melons, and pears.

Lean Meat and Seafood

The key word here is lean. These types of meats are low in fat and high in protein. Some examples of these foods are seafood, turkey, and chicken. Cooking them by grilling, poaching, and baking is best. Always avoid frying.

Egg Whites

The entire egg is filled with nutrients and protein, but the yolk is also high in fat. This could trigger acid reflux. Sticking to just the whites is a great way to get in the protein without the added fat.

Healthy Fats

Good fats can actually help with acid reflux. It is the saturated and trans fats that cause a significant problem. While it is not good to eat large amounts of any fat, healthy fats are packed full of nutrients and can help lessen the symptoms of acid reflux. Sources of healthy fats include avocados, nuts, flaxseed, and olive oil.

What to Drink

We already know that drinks high in caffeine, highly acidic drinks, and carbonated drinks are not good for acid reflux. However, we haven't spoken about the types of drinks that you should consume. Do not overlook this. Now you should not be drinking too many liquids, as this could cause your acid reflux to flare up, but many drinks are very good for you.

Herbal Teas

Herbal teas are great for aiding digestion and are used for various digestive problems. Chamomile, licorice, and ginger teas are the best for acid reflux. They calm the stomach and can help in soothing you. Just remember to avoid mint teas.

Smoothies

These are definitely a great way to get added nutrients into your diet. The best part is that you can add ingredients that will help in soothing your heartburn. Bananas, apples, ginger, and non-citrus fruits are all great options. Smoothies are easy to digest, easy to swallow, and are very cooling when they go down. Having a smoothie with the right ingredients can help with acid reflux and its symptoms.

Fruit Juices

We have already spoken about avoiding citrus fruits in your diet, but citrus fruits are not the only fruits that make great juices. There are plenty of non-citrus fruits that can be juiced. One of the best habits to get your fruit juice is cold-pressed juices. These retain their nutrients and are free from unnecessary ingredients and flavorings. You can buy them in the shops or buy a juicer and juice your own fruits and veggies. Some great options are carrot, ginger, aloe Vera, watermelon, and cucumber.

Water

We should all be getting enough water into our diets. The PH of the water is neutral, which means it can help raise the PH of an acidic meal. Drinking too much water can have adverse effects on acid reflux, so don't overdo it. If you drink when you are thirsty, you should be fine.

Food Swaps

Food swaps are one of the best ways to transition into a new diet or way of eating. We all have our favorites, and sometimes it can be hard to give certain things up. Food swapping allows you to use something similar in the place of the food or ingredients you love. Let's take a look at some food swaps you can make in your everyday life.

Coffee for Herbal Tea

There are many coffee drinkers out there, but unfortunately, caffeine makes it bad for those who suffer from acid reflux. If you still want a nice warm drink, try going for herbal teas instead. They are much easier on the stomach, and many of them actually aid in digestion. You can add some milk to it for a creamier drink if you are not happy with just the tea and water. Once you get used to drinking tea, you won't even miss the coffee. It is just a matter of pushing through until you no longer crave coffee. Remember that caffeine is addictive, and that is why so many people struggle to give up coffee. If you are someone who has coffee multiple times a day, then you might have to either wean yourself off it or suffer from a few withdrawal symptoms before you can go without it. Don't be disheartened if it is a bit hard at the beginning. You will eventually not even miss it.

Citrus Fruit for Berries and Melons

The reason so many people love citrus fruit is that they are so juicy and sweet. Fortunately, there are plenty of other fruits that have the same characteristics. They may not taste the same, but melons and berries are juicy and delicious. Fill your fridge and fruit basket with these fruits instead of citrus fruits.

I would go as far as to say that berries and melons are much better than citrus fruits in terms of variety and usability. You can cook with berries much easier and transform them into your dishes. Using them as garnishes and toppings is also a great idea. Smoothies with these fruits are also super delicious. The possibilities are endless.

Chocolate for Carob Powder or Alkalized Cocoa

I think giving up chocolate is one that makes many people who suffer from acid reflux very sad. Almost everyone enjoys a block of chocolate. The thing is that chocolate is both high in fat and acidic. That is a double trigger, which is why it is best just to give it a skip if you suffer from acid reflux. If you can have a block now without it triggering heartburn, then, by all means, go for it. Just be careful and don't overdo it.

If you really need a chocolate fix, then try carob powder or alkalized cocoa. Alkalized cocoa is also called Dutch-processed powder and is more alkaline than acidic. This makes it safe for people who suffer from acid reflux. Carob powder is not related to cocoa at all and comes from the carob pod. It has very similar flavors to cocoa and you can use it in any recipe that asks for cocoa.

However, it is not a smart idea to just grab a spoonful of these powders and eat it straight. They will have a very bitter taste. You need to add them to the dishes. Chocolate cakes and desserts can be made using either of these two, and that should satisfy your chocolate cravings.

Fried Food for Baked Food

Fried food is generally bad for everyone, even if they don't suffer from acid reflux. The high-fat content is a massive contributor to weight gain, and it is also a trigger for acid reflux. It is best to give fried foods a skip and try and cut it out of your diet as much as you can.

You can bake basically anything that you can fry. Since it is the method of cooking that is changing here, you don't have to change the actual foods you are eating. There are plenty of recipes out there that turn regular foods into healthy, baked alternatives.

High-Fat Dairy for Plant-Based Options

Dairy products are also a common acid reflux trigger. Again, this can be a hard one for people to give up since it seems almost to be a staple in everybody's home. The good news is that there are plenty of plant-based dairy alternatives. These are easy to get at supermarkets, and many of them are not too expensive either.

Milk alternatives are soy milk, almond milk, and oat milk. Instead of regular yogurt, go for coconut yogurt. You can use all of these as direct substitutes for typical dairy products. Therefore, it makes it easy to add to your favorite recipes. If you are looking for a cheese substitute, you can get vegan cheese. It is more expensive than regular cheese. But if you want a sprinkle of cheese, it is an option. You can also add a bit of nutritional yeast for a cheesy flavor to your meal.

Tomato Pasta Sauce for Pesto

Tomato sauces on pasta are classic, but that is not the only way to enjoy pasta. Pesto is a great way to eat pasta, and it is delicious. You could also use some olive oil over your pasta for a simpler dish. Pasta is great with many things, so don't feel stuck because you are giving the red sauce a skip. You could also try making the low-acid tomato sauce recipes in this book if you are craving some tomato paste. It is a great way to enjoy the red sauce too. Again, just be careful not to overdo it, since not all the acid will be neutralized.

Garlic and Onions for Dried Versions

Although never eaten on their own, these two add a lot of flavors to food. Many dishes require one or both, so it can be difficult to get a flavorful dish without them. Instead of using fresh garlic and onions, try the dried variety. They are less likely to cause acid reflux. The other bonus is that you don't always have to be chopping onions or crushing garlic when you are making a meal.

There is a chance that the dried variety might still be a trigger for you. If this is the case, try using other herbs and spices for flavor. Basil, dill, and parsley add a lot of flavors to a variety of dishes. None of them taste like garlic or onion, but that does not mean that you won't be able to get a delicious-tasting meal using them.

Alcohol for Non-Alcoholic Alternatives

Unfortunately, alcohol is a big acid reflux trigger, so it is best to avoid it altogether. If you are slightly tolerant, you can perhaps have one drink. However, be sure not to overdo it. It is important to know your limits as your health is the most important thing.

Thankfully, if you enjoy having a drink on certain occasions, there are alcohol-free options for you. You should still avoid carbonated beverages, so it will still not be a good idea to have non-alcoholic champagne and non-alcoholic beer. Rather, enjoy non-alcoholic wines and mocktails (which taste just like regular cocktails, but without the alcohol). In any case, you don't need alcohol in your life. It isn't a staple, so don't feel like you are missing out because you can't have a drink.

CAPITOLO 11:

21-Day Food Plan to Rest the Digestive System

Day	Breakfast	Lunch	Dinner	Desserts
1	Honeyed Mini Corn Muffins	Seafood Paella Recipe	Lean Spring Stew	Vanilla Pudding
2	Buttermilk Biscuits	Sicilian Seafood Stew	Yummy Chicken Bites	Maple-Ginger Pudding
3	Baked Tortilla Chips with Black Bean Dip	Seafood Stew	Shrimp Scampi	Pumpkin-Maple Custard
4	Jicama With Low-Fat Ranch Dip	Fritto Misto With Gremolata	Zucchini Frittata	Gingered Red Applesauce
5	Baked Green Bean "Fries" With French Fry Sauce	Fritto Misto	Salmon Patties	Ginger-Berry Yogurt Pops
6	Maple-Thyme Roasted Carrots	Fish Soup	Stuff Cheese Pork Chops	Bananas With Maple Brown Sugar Sauce
7	Roasted Parmesan Potatoes	Chicken Chasseur	Italian Pork Chops	Honey-Cinnamon Poached Pears
8	Quick Rice Pilaf	Smoky Chicken Traybake	Sunshine Wrap	Baked Red Apples
9	Mushroom And Pea Couscous	Chicken And Orzo Bake	Taco Omelet	Froyo With Blueberry Sauce
10	Simple Sautéed Greens	One-Pot Roast	Sheet Pan Spicy Tofu and Green Beans	Flourless Peanut Butter Cookies
11	Avocado Deviled Eggs	Beef Curry	Skillet Chicken Thighs with Potato, Apple, And Spinach	Mixed Berry Popsicles
12	Roasted Fennel	Beef Schnitzel	Cherry Tomatoes Tilapia Salad	Chocolate Avocado Pudding
13	No-Fat Biscuits	Beef Massaman Curry	Apple Cider Glazed Chicken Breast with Carrots	Instant Frozen Berry Yogurt
14	Easy Cornbread	Barbecued Rump of Beef in Dijon	Onion Paprika Pork Tenderloin	Chocolate Protein Balls
15	Shredded Brussels Sprouts	Roast Rib of Beef	Rosemary Garlic Pork Chops	Mozzarella Balls Recipe
16	Maple-Ginger Roasted Beets	Beef Wellington with Stilton	Skinny Chicken Pesto Bake	Strawberry Frozen Yogurt
17	Ginger Mashed Sweet Potatoes	Marinated Lamb Steaks	Cold Tomato Couscous	Chocolate Protein Pudding Pops
18	Calm Carrot Salad	Lamb Kofta Curry	Fresh Shrimp Rolls	Red Energy Wonders
19	Zucchini Hummus	Mediterranean Lamb Stew with Olives	Chicken Breast Tortilla	Chocolate Almond Ginger Mousse
20	Playgroup Granola Bars	Herb And Spiced Lamb	Veggie Quesadillas with Cilantro Yogurt Dip	Peanut Butter Joy Cookies
21	Zucchini And Salmon Canapés	Miso Soup with Tofu and Greens	Mayo-Less Tuna Salad	Sweet Pumpkin Pudding

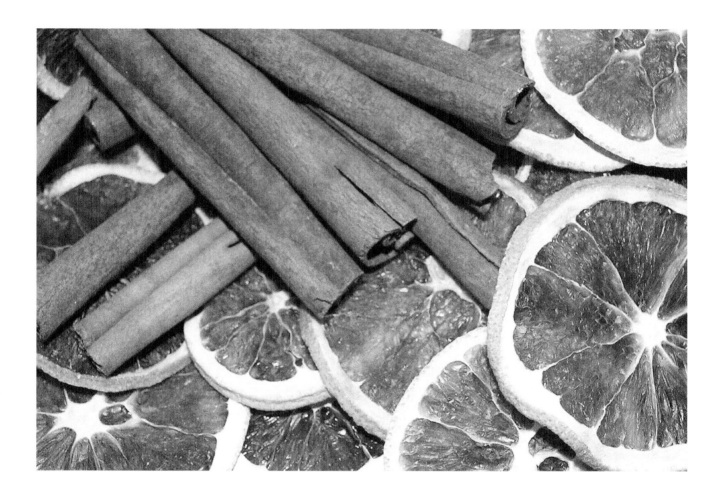

CAPITOLO 12:

Appetizers for the Health of the Gastric Walls

1.   Cinnamon Apple "Fries"

Preparation Time: 10 minutes
Cooking Time: 12 minutes
Servings: 4
Ingredients:

- 2 red apples, peeled, cored, and cut into wedges
- 1 tbsp. melted coconut oil
- 1 tbsp. pure maple syrup
- 1 tsp. ground cinnamon
- A pinch sea salt

Directions:

1. Preheat the oven to 375°F.
2. Line a baking sheet with parchment paper.
3. In a large bowl, toss together the apples, coconut oil, maple syrup, cinnamon, and salt until evenly coated. Spread the apples in a single layer on the prepared sheet.
4. Bake for about 12 minutes, or until the apples are browned.

Nutrition:

- Calories: 98
- Fats: 2 g
- Saturated Fat: 2 g
- Cholesterol: 8 mg
- Carbs: 19 g
- Fiber: 3 g
- Protein: <1 g
- Sodium: 61 mg

2.   Bacon-Wrapped Melon

Preparation Time: 10 minutes
Cooking Time: 0 minutes
Servings: 4
Ingredients:

- ½ cantaloupe, rind removed and seeded, cut into 8 wedges
- 8 very thin Canadian bacon slices

Directions:

1. Wrap each melon wedge with 1 piece of Canadian bacon, and secure them with a toothpick.

Nutrition:

- Calories: 28
- Fats: 1 g
- Saturated Fat: 0 g
- Cholesterol: 7 mg
- Carbs: 2 g
- Fiber: 0 g
- Protein: 3 g
- Sodium: 302 mg

3. Honeyed Mini Corn Muffins

Preparation Time: 5 minutes
Cooking Time: 15 minutes
Servings: 12
Ingredients:

- 1 ¾ cups cornmeal
- ¾ cup all-purpose flour
- 1 tbsp. baking powder
- 1 tsp. baking soda
- ¼ tsp. sea salt
- 1½ cups unsweetened almond milk
- ¼ cup honey
- 2 eggs, beaten
- 2 tbsp. canola oil
- 2 tbsp. nonfat plain Greek-style yogurt

Directions:

1. Preheat the oven to 425°F.
2. Line a 24-cup mini muffin tin with mini cupcake liners.
3. In a medium bowl, whisk the cornmeal, flour, baking powder, baking soda, and salt together.
4. In another medium bowl, whisk together the almond milk, honey, eggs, oil, and yogurt.
5. Add the wet ingredients to the dry ingredients and mix until just combined. Fill each muffin cup ½ to ¾ full.
6. Bake for about 15 minutes, or until a toothpick inserted in the center comes out clean.

Nutrition:

- Calories: 217
- Fats: 11 g
- Saturated Fat: 7 g
- Cholesterol: 27 mg
- Carbs: 28 g
- Fiber: 2 g
- Protein: 4 g
- Sodium: 167 mg

4. Buttermilk Biscuits

Preparation Time: 15 minutes
Cooking Time: 15 minutes
Servings: 8
Ingredients:

- ¾ cup all-purpose flour
- ¾ cup whole wheat flour
- 1 tsp. baking soda
- ½ tsp. sea salt
- 2 tbsp. cold unsalted butter, cut into small pieces
- ½ cup nonfat plain Greek-style yogurt
- ¼ cup low-fat buttermilk
- 2 tbsp. honey

Directions:

1. Preheat the oven to 425°F.
2. Line a baking sheet with parchment paper.
3. In a medium bowl, whisk together the flours, baking soda, and salt.
4. Using two knives or a pastry blender, cut in the butter until the mixture resembles coarse oatmeal.
5. Stir in the yogurt, buttermilk, and honey.
6. Drop the dough in 8 equal portions onto the prepared sheet. Shape them lightly into rounds.
7. Bake for 14 to 15 minutes, or until golden brown.

Nutrition:

- Calories: 138
- Fats: 3 g
- Saturated Fat: 2 g
- Cholesterol: 8 mg
- Carbs: 24 g
- Fiber: <1 g
- Protein: 4 g
- Sodium: 317 mg

5.   Baked Tortilla Chips with Black Bean Dip

Preparation Time: 10 minutes
Cooking Time: 15 minutes
Servings: 4
Ingredients:

- 4 corn tortillas, cut into 8 wedges each
- 1 tsp. sea salt, divided
- 1 (14-oz.) can black beans, drained and rinsed
- 1 tsp. ground cumin
- ½ tsp. ground coriander
- 2 tbsp. fresh cilantro, chopped

Directions:

1. Preheat the oven to 350°F.
2. Line a baking sheet with parchment paper.
3. Spread the tortilla wedges in a single layer on the prepared sheet. Sprinkle with ¼ teaspoon of salt.
4. Bake for about 15 minutes.
5. Meanwhile, in a medium saucepan over medium-high heat, warm the black beans, cumin, coriander, and the remaining ¾ teaspoon of salt for 5 minutes, stirring occasionally.
6. Transfer the mixture to a blender or food processor and process until smooth. Stir in the cilantro and serve with the warm tortilla wedges.

Nutrition:

- Calories: 393
- Fats: 2 g
- Saturated Fat: 0 g
- Cholesterol: 0 mg
- Carbs: 73 g
- Fiber: 16 g
- Protein: 23 g
- Sodium: 485 mg

6.   Jicama with Low-Fat Ranch Dip

Preparation Time: 10 minutes
Cooking Time: 0 minutes
Servings: 8
Ingredients:

- 1 cup fat-free cottage cheese
- 1 cup fat-free sour cream
- 2 tbsp. fresh dill, chopped
- 1 tbsp. fresh thyme, chopped
- 1 tsp. fresh chives, chopped
- 1 tsp. lemon zest, grated
- ½ tsp. sea salt
- 1 jicama, peeled and sliced

Directions:

1. In a medium bowl, stir together the cottage cheese, sour cream, dill, thyme, chives, lemon zest, and salt. Serve with the sliced jicama for dipping.

Nutrition:

- Calories: 90
- Fats: <1 g
- Saturated Fat: 0 g
- Cholesterol: 5 mg
- Carbs: 14 g
- Fiber: 4 g
- Protein: 6 g
- Sodium: 262 mg

7. Baked Green Bean "Fries" with French Fry Sauce

Preparation Time: 10 minutes
Cooking Time: 15 minutes
Servings: 4
Ingredients:

- Nonstick cooking spray
- ¾ cup bread crumbs
- 1 tsp. dried thyme
- ½ tsp. dried rosemary
- ½ tsp. sea salt
- ¼ tsp. ground cumin
- 2 eggs, beaten
- 1 tsp. Dijon mustard
- 1 lb. fresh green beans, trimmed and halved
- 1 cup French fry sauce

Directions:

1. Preheat the oven to 425°F.
2. Spray a baking sheet with nonstick cooking spray.
3. In a large bowl, mix the bread crumbs, thyme, rosemary, salt, and cumin.
4. In another large bowl, whisk the eggs and mustard together.
5. Add the green beans to the egg mixture and stir to coat.
6. Toss the coated beans with the bread crumbs to coat. Place them in a single layer on the prepared sheet.
7. Bake for about 12 minutes, or until golden brown. Flip and bake for 3 minutes more. Serve with the dipping sauce.

Nutrition:

- Calories: 100
- Fats: 2 g
- Saturated Fat: <1 g
- Cholesterol: 43 mg
- Carbs: 13 g
- Fiber: 3 g
- Protein: 8 g
- Sodium: 607 mg

8. Baked Potato Chips

Preparation Time: 5 minutes
Cooking Time: 25 minutes
Servings: 4
Ingredients:

- Nonstick cooking spray
- 1 medium russet potato, cut into ¼-inch-thick slices
- 2 tbsp. extra-virgin olive oil
- ½ tsp. sea salt

Directions:

1. Preheat the oven to 400°F.
2. Spray a baking sheet with nonstick cooking spray.
3. In a large bowl, mix the potato slices, oil, and salt to coat. Spread the chips in a single layer on the prepared sheet.
4. Bake for about 25 minutes, or until crisp and brown.

Nutrition:

- Calories: 131
- Fats: 7 g
- Saturated Fat: 1 g
- Cholesterol: 0 mg
- Carbs: 16 g
- Fiber: 2 g
- Protein: 2 g
- Sodium: 237 mg

9.   Sweet Potato Oven "Fries"

Preparation Time: 5 minutes
Cooking Time: 25 minutes
Servings: 4
Ingredients:
- Nonstick cooking spray
- 1 medium sweet potato, cut into ¼-inch-thick strips
- 2 tbsp. extra-virgin olive oil
- ½ tsp. sea salt

Directions:
1. Preheat the oven to 450°F.
2. Spray a baking sheet with nonstick cooking spray.
3. In a large bowl, mix the sweet potato strips, oil, and salt to coat. Spread the fries in a single layer on the prepared sheet.
4. Bake for about 25 minutes, or until crisp and brown.

Nutrition:
- Calories: 101
- Fats: 7 g
- Saturated Fat: 1 g
- Cholesterol: 0 mg
- Carbs: 9 g
- Fiber: 2 g
- Protein: <1 g
- Sodium: 244 mg

10.   Maple-Thyme   Roasted Carrots

Preparation Time: 10 minutes
Cooking Time: 20 minutes
Servings: 4
Ingredients:
- Nonstick cooking spray
- 4 carrots, peeled and cut lengthwise into quarters
- 2 tbsp. extra-virgin olive oil
- 1 tsp. orange zest, grated
- ½ tsp. sea salt
- ½ tsp. dried thyme
- 2 tbsp. pure maple syrup

Directions:
1. Preheat the oven to 400°F.
2. Spray a baking sheet with nonstick cooking spray.
3. In a large bowl, mix the carrots, oil, orange zest, salt, and thyme to coat. Spread the carrots in a single layer on the prepared sheet.
4. Bake for about 20 minutes, or until the carrots are brown and roasted.
5. Toss with the maple syrup before serving.

Nutrition:
- Calories: 118
- Fats: 7 g
- Saturated Fat: 1 g
- Cholesterol: 0 mg
- Carbs: 15 g
- Fiber: 2 g
- Protein: <1 g
- Sodium: 277 mg

11.   Roasted Parmesan Potatoes

Preparation Time: 10 minutes
Cooking Time: 20 minutes
Servings: 4
Ingredients:

- Nonstick cooking spray
- 2 cups Yukon Gold potatoes, diced ½-inch pieces
- 2 tbsp. extra-virgin olive oil
- ½ tsp. sea salt
- 1 tbsp. fresh rosemary, chopped
- 2 tbsp. Parmesan cheese, grated

Directions:

1. Preheat the oven to 450°F.
2. Spray a baking sheet with nonstick cooking spray.
3. In a large bowl, mix the potatoes, oil, salt, and rosemary to coat. Place the potatoes in a single layer on the prepared sheet.
4. Bake for about 20 minutes, or until crisp and brown.
5. Toss with the Parmesan cheese before serving.

Nutrition:

- Calories: 113
- Fats: 7 g
- Saturated Fat: 1 g
- Cholesterol: 0 mg
- Carbs: 12 g
- Fiber: 1 g
- Protein: 1 g
- Sodium: 271 mg

12.   Mac 'n' Cheese

Preparation Time: 15 minutes
Cooking Time: 5 minutes
Servings: 4
Ingredients:

- 3 cups (1 recipe) low-fat white sauce
- 2 oz. fat-free sharp Cheddar cheese, grated
- 6 oz. whole wheat elbow macaroni, cooked according to package directions and drained
- 1 tbsp. melted unsalted butter
- ¼ cup bread crumbs

Directions:

1. Preheat the broiler to high.
2. In a medium saucepan over medium heat, cook the white sauce and Cheddar cheese for 2 to 3 minutes, whisking constantly until the cheese melts.
3. Add the hot macaroni and toss to coat. Divide evenly among four (6-oz.) ramekins, or spread into a baking dish.
4. In a small bowl, mix the butter and bread crumbs. Sprinkle over the mac 'n' cheese.
5. Broil for 1 to 2 minutes, or until the bread crumbs are golden brown.

Nutrition:

- Calories: 258
- Fats: 5 g
- Saturated Fat: 2 g
- Cholesterol: 14 mg
- Carbs: 41 g
- Fiber: 4 g
- Protein: 12 g
- Sodium: 343 mg

13.   Quick Rice Pilaf

Preparation Time: 10 minutes
Cooking Time: 10 minutes
Servings: 4
Ingredients:

- 2 tbsp. extra-virgin olive oil
- 1 carrot, peeled and cut into ¼-inch dice
- ½ apple, peeled and cut into ¼-inch dice
- ¼ cup slivered almonds
- 1 tsp. dried thyme
- ½ tsp. sea salt
- 1 cup cooked brown rice
- ¼ cup vegetable broth

Directions:

1. In a large sauté pan or skillet over medium-high heat, heat the oil until it shimmers.
2. Add the carrot, apple, almonds, thyme, and salt. Cook for about 5 minutes, stirring occasionally until the apples and carrots are soft.
3. Stir in the rice and broth. Cook for 5 minutes more, stirring occasionally.

Nutrition:

- Calories: 290
- Fats: 11 g
- Saturated Fat: 2 g
- Cholesterol: 0 mg
- Carbs: 43 g
- Fiber: 4 g
- Protein: 5 g
- Sodium: 295 mg

14.   Mushroom and Pea Couscous

Preparation Time: 10 minutes
Cooking Time: 5 minutes
Servings: 4
Ingredients:

- 1 tbsp. extra-virgin olive oil
- 1 cup sliced mushrooms
- 1 cup peas, fresh or frozen
- 1½ cups vegetable broth
- ½ tsp. dried thyme
- ¼ tsp. sea salt
- 1 cup couscous

Directions:

1. In a medium pot over medium-high heat, heat the oil until it shimmers.
2. Add the mushrooms and cook for 5 minutes, stirring occasionally.
3. Add the peas, broth, thyme, and salt. Bring to a boil.
4. Remove from the heat and stir in the couscous. Cover and let sit for 10 minutes. Fluff with a fork.

Nutrition:

- Calories: 240
- Fats: 5 g
- Saturated Fat: <1 g
- Cholesterol: 0 mg
- Carbs: 40 g
- Fiber: 4 g
- Protein: 10 g
- Sodium: 410 mg

15.   Simple Sautéed Greens

Preparation Time: 5 minutes
Cooking Time: 10 minutes
Servings: 4
Ingredients:

- 2 tbsp. extra-virgin olive oil
- 4 cups chopped kale, or other green of choice
- 2 tbsp. vegetable broth
- 1 lemon, zested
- ½ tsp. sea salt
- A pinch ground nutmeg

Directions:

1. In a 10- or 12-inch sauté pan or skillet over medium-high heat, heat the oil until it shimmers.
2. Add the kale, broth, and lemon zest. Cook for 5 to 10 minutes, stirring constantly until the kale is very soft.
3. Season with the salt and nutmeg. Serve immediately.

Nutrition:

- Calories: 95
- Fats: 7 g
- Saturated Fat: 1 g
- Cholesterol: 0 mg
- Carbs: 7 g
- Fiber: 1 g
- Protein: 2 g
- Sodium: 287 mg

16.   Mixed Veggie Stir-Fry

Preparation Time: 5 minutes
Cooking Time: 6 minutes
Servings: 4
Ingredients:

- 2 tbsp. extra-virgin olive oil
- 1 cup mushrooms, sliced
- 1 cup peas, fresh or frozen
- 1 carrot, peeled and diced
- 1 cup broccoli florets
- ½ tsp. ground ginger
- 2 tbsp. gluten-free soy sauce

Directions:

1. In a 10- or 12-inch sauté pan or skillet over medium-high heat, heat the oil until it shimmers.
2. Add the mushrooms, peas, carrot, broccoli, and ginger. Cook for about 5 minutes, stirring frequently until the veggies are soft.
3. Stir in the soy sauce. Simmer for 1 minute more.

Nutrition:

- Calories: 110
- Fats: 7 g
- Saturated Fat: 1 g
- Cholesterol: 0 mg
- Carbs: 10 g
- Fiber: 3 g
- Protein: 3 g
- Sodium: 499 mg

17. Guacamole

Preparation Time: 10 minutes
Cooking Time: 0 minutes
Servings: 6
Ingredients:

- 2 avocados, peeled, pitted, and chopped
- ¼ cup fresh cilantro, chopped
- 2 tbsp. fat-free plain Greek yogurt
- ½ tsp. ground cumin
- ½ tsp. lime zest, grated
- ½ tsp. sea salt, or to taste

Directions:

1. Combine all the ingredients in a medium bowl. Mash and mix with a fork until the avocados are mashed and the ingredients are well blended.

Nutrition:

- Calories: 101
- Fats: 9 g
- Sodium: 202 mg
- Carbs: 5 g
- Fiber: 4 g
- Protein: 2 g

18. Avocado Deviled Eggs

Preparation Time: 10 minutes
Cooking Time: 0 minutes
Servings: 4
Ingredients:

- 4 large hardboiled eggs, peeled and sliced in half lengthwise
- 2 tbsp. fat-free plain Greek yogurt
- ½ avocado, peeled, pitted, and mashed
- 1 tsp. orange zest
- ¼ cup fresh tarragon, chopped
- ½ tsp. sea salt

Directions:

1. Use a spoon to scoop the egg yolks from the whites. Put the egg yolks in a small bowl and put the whites cut-side up on a platter.
2. Add the yogurt, avocado, orange zest, tarragon, and salt to the egg yolks. Mash with a fork and mix.
3. Spoon or pipe the mixture into the egg halves.

Nutrition:

- Calories: 123
- Fats: 9 g
- Sodium: 358 mg
- Carbs: 4 g
- Fiber: 2 g
- Protein: 8 g

19. Roasted Fennel

Preparation Time: 10 minutes
Cooking Time: 40 minutes
Servings: 4
Ingredients:

- 2 fennel bulbs, cored and cut into pieces
- 2 tbsp. olive oil
- ½ tsp. sea salt
- ½ tsp. grated lemon zest

Directions:

1. Preheat the oven to 400°F.
2. In a large bowl, toss the fennel with the olive oil and salt. Spread in an even layer on a rimmed baking sheet.
3. Bake until the fennel begins to brown, about 40 minutes, flipping after about 20 minutes.
4. Toss with the lemon zest before serving.

Nutrition:

- Calories: 96
- Fats: 7 g
- Sodium: 352 mg
- Carbs: 9 g
- Fiber: 4 g
- Protein: 2 g

20. Honey-Roasted Carrots

Preparation Time: 4 minutes
Cooking Time: 40 minutes
Servings: 40
Ingredients:

- 2 cups baby carrots, halved lengthwise
- 2 tbsp. olive oil
- ¼ cup honey
- ½ tsp. sea salt

Directions:

1. Preheat the oven to 400°F.
2. In a large bowl, toss the carrots with the olive oil, honey, and salt. Place in a single layer on a baking sheet.
3. Bake until the carrots soften and begin to brown, about 40 minutes, flipping after about 20 minutes.

Nutrition:

- Calories: 142
- Fats: 7 g
- Sodium: 322 mg
- Carbs: 22 g
- Fiber: 1 g
- Protein: 1 g

21.   No-Fat Biscuits

Preparation Time: 10 minutes
Cooking Time: 25 minutes
Servings: 6
Ingredients:

- Nonstick cooking spray
- 2 cups all-purpose flour
- ¾ tsp. baking soda
- 2 tsp. baking powder
- A pinch sea salt
- 1 ¼ cups nonfat plain yogurt

Directions:

1. Preheat the oven to 425°F. Spray a rimmed baking sheet with nonstick cooking spray.
2. In a medium bowl, whisk together the flour, baking soda, baking powder, and salt.
3. Fold in the yogurt until just mixed.
4. Use a large spoon to form 6 biscuits on the prepared baking sheet.
5. Bake until the biscuits are golden brown, about 20 to 25 minutes.

Nutrition:

- Calories: 161 Fats: 0 g
- Sodium: 373 mg Carbs: 34 g
- Fiber: 1 g Protein: 7 g

22.   Easy Cornbread

Preparation Time: 20 minutes
Cooking Time: 20 minutes
Servings: 6
Ingredients:

- Nonstick cooking spray
- ¾ cup all-purpose flour
- 1 ½ cups cornmeal
- 1 tbsp. baking powder
- ¼ tsp. sea salt
- 1 large egg, beaten
- 1 cup nonfat milk

Directions:

1. Preheat the oven to 425°F. Spray a 9-inch baking pan with nonstick cooking spray.
2. In a medium bowl, whisk together the flour, cornmeal, baking powder, and salt.
3. In a small bowl, whisk together the egg and milk.
4. Add the wet ingredients to the dry ingredients and fold together until just combined. Pour into the prepared pan.
5. Bake until browned, about 20 minutes.

Nutrition:

- Calories: 188 Fats: 2 g
- Sodium: 380 mg Carbs: 37 g
- Fiber: 3 g Protein: 6 g

23.   Shredded Brussels Sprouts

Preparation Time: 10 minutes
Cooking Time: 7 minutes
Servings: 4
Ingredients:

- 1 tbsp. olive oil
- 8 ounces Brussels sprouts, shredded or julienned
- ½ tsp. sea salt

Directions:

1. Place a large nonstick skillet over medium-high heat and add the olive oil. Once the oil is shimmering, add the Brussels sprouts and salt. Cook, stirring occasionally until the sprouts are browned, about 5 to 7 minutes.

Nutrition:

- Calories: 54
- Fats: 4 g
- Sodium: 305 mg
- Carbs: 5 g
- Fiber: 2 g
- Protein: 2 g

24.   Maple-Ginger Roasted Beets

Preparation Time: 10 minutes
Cooking Time: 1 hour
Servings: 4
Ingredients:

- 8 oz. beets, peeled and quartered
- 2 tbsp. olive oil
- ½ tsp. sea salt
- 1 tbsp. fresh ginger, grated
- ¼ cup pure maple syrup

Directions:

1. Preheat the oven to 400°F.
2. Place the beets on a rimmed baking sheet and drizzle with the olive oil. Toss to coat. Sprinkle with the salt and ginger.
3. Roast for 30 minutes. Remove from the oven. Drizzle the beets with the syrup and stir to mix. Return to the oven and continue roasting for 30 minutes more.

Nutrition:

- Calories: 137
- Fats: 7 g
- Sodium: 337 mg
- Carbs: 19 g
- Fiber: 2 g
- Protein: 1 g

25. Ginger-Cumin Kale Chips

Preparation Time: 10 minutes
Cooking Time: 20 minutes
Servings: 6
Ingredients:

- 1 bunch kale, stems removed and leaves trimmed
- 1 tbsp. olive oil
- ½ tsp. sea salt
- 1 tbsp. fresh ginger, grated
- ½ tsp. ground cumin

Directions:

1. Preheat the oven to 350°F. Line a rimmed baking sheet with parchment paper.
2. In a large bowl, toss the kale leaves with the olive oil, salt, ginger, and cumin.
3. Spread in an even layer on the prepared baking pan.
4. Bake until the kale is crisp and starting to brown, about 20 minutes, flipping after about 10 minutes.

Nutrition:

- Calories: 40 Fats: 3 g
- Sodium: 209 mg Carbs: 4 g
- Fiber: 1 g Protein: 1 g

26. Ginger Mashed Sweet Potatoes

Preparation Time: 10 minutes
Cooking Time: 15 minutes
Servings: 4
Ingredients:

- 2 sweet potatoes, peeled and cut into 1-inch pieces
- 2 cups water
- 1 tbsp. fresh ginger, grated
- ½ cup nonfat milk or nondairy milk
- ¼ cup nonfat plain yogurt
- ½ tsp. sea salt

Directions:

1. Place the sweet potatoes in a large pot and cover with at least 2 inches of water. Place over medium-high heat and bring to a boil.
2. Cover and cook until the potatoes are tender, about 15 minutes.
3. Drain the potatoes and return them to the pot. Add the ginger, milk, yogurt, and salt.
4. Mash with a potato masher until smooth, and then stir well to combine.

Nutrition:

- Calories: 87 Fats: <1 g
- Sodium: 322 mg Carbs: 19 g
- Fiber: 2 g Protein: 3 g

27. Calm Carrot Salad

Preparation Time: 10 minutes
Cooking Time: 0 minutes
Servings: 2
Ingredients:

- 2 tbsp. Splenda®
- 2 tbsp. raisins
- 2 tsp. olive oil
- ¼ tsp. salt
- ¼ lb. mesclun greens
- 1 lb. carrots, trimmed and grated
- 1 tsp. dried oregano

Directions:

1. Mix oregano, Splenda®, salt, raisins, and olive oil in a medium bowl.
2. Toss in the carrots and mix well to coat.
3. Adjust the seasoning with salt.
4. Serve over the mesclun greens.

Nutrition:

- Calories: 144
- Fats: 0.4 g
- Carbs: 8 g
- Protein: 5.6 g

28. Millet Cauliflower Mash

Preparation Time: 10 minutes
Cooking Time: 30 minutes
Servings: 4
Ingredients:

- 1 tsp. tamari
- 3 cups water
- 1 cup cauliflower florets
- 2 tsp. parsley sprig
- 1 cup millet
- ¼ tsp. salt

Directions:

1. Roast the millet in a nonstick pan for 5 minutes.
2. Boil the water in a large pan on high heat, then add the cauliflower, salt, and millet.
3. Cover the dish with the lid, then cook for 25 minutes on low heat.
4. Stir in the tamari and cook for 5 minutes.
5. Lightly mash the cauliflower mixture.
6. Garnish with parsley and serve.

Nutrition:

- Calories: 454
- Fats: 4 g
- Carbs: 30 g
- Protein: 4 g

29.   Spinach and Dill Dip

Preparation Time: 5 minutes
Cooking Time: 3 minutes
Servings: 4
Ingredients:

- 2 cups baby spinach
- ½ tsp. lemon zest, grated
- ¼ tsp. sea salt
- 1 cup lactose-free nonfat plain yogurt
- 2 tbsp. fresh dill, chopped

Directions:

1. In a large nonstick skillet, add the spinach, lemon zest, and sea salt. Cook, stirring, until the spinach wilts, 2 to 3 minutes. Remove from the heat and allow the spinach to cool.
2. In a small bowl, combine the cooled spinach, yogurt, and dill, stirring to combine.
3. Serve.

Nutrition:

- Calories: 68
- Protein: 4 g
- Fats: 4 g
- Carbs: 5 g

30.   Zucchini Hummus

Preparation Time: 5 minutes
Cooking Time: 0 minutes
Servings: 4
Ingredients:

- 1 medium zucchini, chopped
- 1 tbsp. olive oil
- 1 tbsp. tahini
- 1 tsp. fresh dill, chopped
- ½ tsp. lemon zest, grated
- ½ tsp. sea salt

Directions:

1. In a blender or food processor, combine all the ingredients. Blend until smooth. Serve.

Nutrition:

- Calories: 60
- Protein: 6 g
- Fats: 3 g
- Carbs: 2 g

31.   Zucchini   and   Salmon Canapés

Preparation Time: 15 minutes
Cooking Time: 0 minutes
Servings: 4
Ingredients:

- 4 oz. canned salmon, drained, rinsed, and flaked
- ¼ cup lactose-free nonfat plain yogurt
- 1 tsp. orange zest, grated
- 1 tsp. fresh tarragon, chopped
- ½ tsp. sea salt
- 1 zucchini, cut into 12 rounds

Directions:

1. In a small bowl, combine the salmon, yogurt, orange zest, tarragon, and salt.
2. Spoon onto the zucchini rounds.
3. Serve.

Nutrition:

- Calories: 53
- Protein: 7 g
- Fats: 2 g
- Carbs: 1 g

32.   Olive Tapenade

Preparation Time: 15 minutes
Cooking Time: 0 minutes
Servings: 4
Ingredients:

- ½ cup black olives, pitted and chopped
- ½ anchovy fillet, chopped
- 1 tbsp. olive oil
- 2 tbsp. fresh basil, chopped
- ½ tsp. lemon zest

Directions:

1. In a small bowl, mix all the ingredients until well combined.
2. Serve.

Nutrition:

- Calories: 51
- Protein: 0 g
- Fats: 5 g
- Carbs: 1 g

33.   Sweet Potato French Fries

Preparation Time: 10 minutes
Cooking Time: 20 minutes
Servings: 2
Ingredients:

- 1 sweet potato, peeled and cut into ¼-inch matchsticks
- 1 tsp. ground cumin
- ½ tsp. sea salt
- 1 tbsp. olive oil

Directions:

1. Preheat the oven to 450°F.
2. In a bowl, toss together the sweet potato sticks, cumin, salt, and olive oil.
3. Spread in a single layer on a rimmed baking sheet.
4. Bake, turning once with a spatula until the fries are browned and tender, about 20 minutes. Serve.

Nutrition:

- Calories: 115
- Protein: 1 g
- Fats: 7 g
- Carbs: 14 g

34.   Chicken Fajita Salad

Preparation Time: 10 minutes
Cooking Time: 5 minutes
Servings: 4
Ingredients:
For the Marinade/Dressing:

- 3 tbsp. olive oil
- 2 tbsp. cilantro, chopped
- 2 cloves garlic, crushed
- 1 tsp. Splenda®
- ¾ tsp. red chili flakes
- ½ tsp. ground Cumin
- 1 tsp. salt

For the Salad:

- 4 chicken thigh fillets, skin removed
- ½ yellow bell pepper, sliced and deseeded
- ½ red bell pepper, deseeded and sliced
- ½ an onion, sliced
- 5 cups Romaine, (or cos) lettuce leaves, washed and dried
- 2 avocados, sliced
- Extra cilantro leaves to garnish
- Sour cream, (optional) to serve

Directions:

1. To make the marinade combine all of its ingredients in a bowl.
2. Season the chicken pieces with this marinade.
3. Marinate the meat in the refrigerator for 2 hours.
4. Heat 1 teaspoon of oil in a grill pan. Sear the chicken from sides until golden brown.
5. Transfer the chicken to a plate.
6. Sauté the onions and the pepper in the same pan.
7. Slice the chicken and toss it with the pepper, onion, avocado, and leaves in a bowl.
8. Stir in the salad dressing.
9. Toss well and serve.

Nutrition:

- Calories: 184
- Fats: 37 g
- Saturated Fat: 8 g
- Cholesterol: 110 mg
- Sodium: 689 mg
- Carbs: 13 g
- Fiber: 8 g
- Sugar: 3 g
- Protein 19 g

35.   Playgroup Granola Bars

Preparation Time: 10 minutes
Cooking Time: 35 minutes
Servings: 4
Ingredients:

- 2 cups rolled oats
- ¾ cup packed coconut sugar
- ½ cup wheat germ
- ¾ tsp. ground cinnamon
- 1 cup almond flour
- ¾ cup raisins (optional)
- ¾ tsp. salt
- ½ cup honey
- 1 egg, beaten
- ½ cup vegetable oil
- 2 tsp. vanilla extract

Directions:

1. Set the oven at 350°F to preheat. Grease a 9x13-inch pan with cooking spray.
2. Toss the oats with the wheat germ, flour, raisins, salt, cinnamon, and coconut sugar in a bowl
3. Add the egg white, oil, vanilla, and honey to the mixture.
4. Mix well with your hands and then transfer it to the baking pan.
5. Bake for 35 minutes, or until golden brown around the edges.
6. Slice and serve.

Nutrition:

- Calories: 307 Fats: 25 g
- Saturated Fat: 5 g Cholesterol: 16 mg
- Sodium: 372 mg Carbs: 16 g
- Fiber: 5 g Sugar: 4 g Protein: 10 g

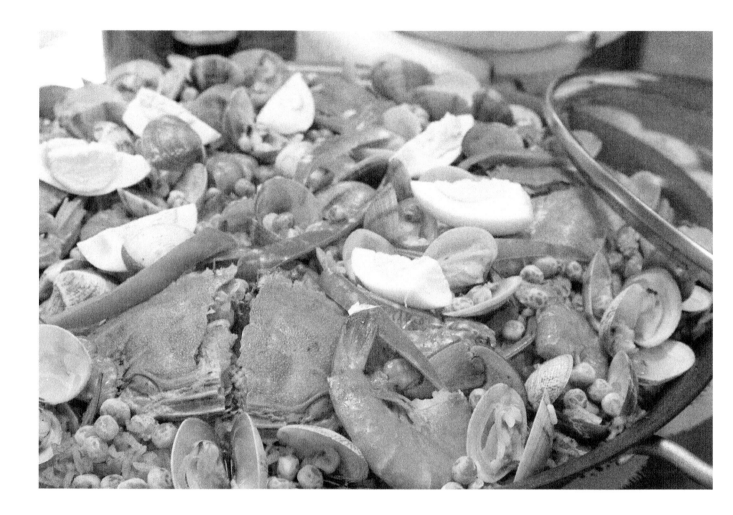

CAPITOLO 13:

First Courses to Reduce Heartburn

1.   Seafood Paella Recipe

Preparation Time: 10 minutes
Cooking Time: 22 minutes
Servings: 4
Ingredients:

- 1 ½-pint fish stock
- A pinch saffron
- 1 ½ tbsp. extra-virgin olive oil
- 1 large onion, finely chopped
- 3 garlic cloves, crushed
- 1 (1 ¼-oz.) pack, flat-leaf parsley, leaves chopped
- 1 tsp. black pepper
- 2 ¼ cups (8-oz.) Spanish paella rice
- 1 cup red bell pepper, chopped
- 2 ¼ cup jars roasted peppers, drain and rinse them
- 1 ⅓ cup (6-oz.) raw black tiger prawns
- 1 ¼ cup (5-oz.) live mussels, cleaned and debearded
- 1 ¼ cup raw squid rings
- 1 lemon, cut into wedges

Directions:

1. Boil the fish stock with saffron and keep it aside.
2. Preheat the oil to sauté the onion for 5 minutes.
3. Add the garlic, bell pepper, parsley, and black pepper. Stir-cook for 2 minutes.
4. Stir in the rice and stock, and cook for 10 minutes.
5. Add in roasted peppers and cook for 5 minutes.
6. Place prawns, mussels, and squid rings in the pan.
7. Cook for 5 minutes, then take off the heat.
8. Cover the pan with foil and let it sit for 5 minutes.
9. Garnish with the parsley.
10. Serve.

Nutrition:

- Calories: 272 Fats: 11 g
- Saturated Fat: 3 g Cholesterol: 66 mg
- Sodium: 288 mg Carbs: 10 g
- Fiber: 4 g
- Sugar: 0 g
- Protein: 33 g

2.   Sicilian Seafood Stew

Preparation Time: 10 minutes
Cooking Time: 20 minutes
Servings: 4
Ingredients:

- 2 tbsp. olive oil
- 1 onion, chopped
- 2 sticks celery, chopped
- 2 garlic cloves, chopped, plus an extra clove
- 1 anchovy, rinsed
- 1 tsp. dried chili flakes
- 1 cup red bell pepper
- ½ cup nonfat yogurt
- 2 cups vegetable stock
- 3 cups raw peeled prawns
- 2 cups new potatoes
- 1 lemon, zested and juiced
- 1 tsp. baby capers
- 1 tsp. flat-leaf parsley, chopped

Directions:

1. Preheat the olive oil in a suitable pot, and sauté the celery, onion, anchovy, garlic, and chili.
2. Season with pepper and salt. Stir-cook for 5 minutes.
3. Meanwhile, boil the potatoes until al dente. Cut them into thick slices.
4. Add the stock, yogurt, and bell pepper to the pan, and cook for 15 minutes.
5. Place the prawns in the pan along with the potatoes, capers, lemon zest, and juice.
6. Cook for 5 minutes and then serve.

Nutrition:

- Calories: 557
- Fats: 29 g Saturated Fat: 22 g
- Cholesterol: 550 mg
- Sodium: 1800 mg
- Carbs: 25 g
- Fiber: 3 g
- Sugar: 0.3 g
- Protein: 47 g

3.   Seafood Stew

Preparation Time: 5 minutes
Cooking Time: 17 minutes
Servings: 4
Ingredients:

- 1 large onion, finely sliced
- 1 garlic clove, finely chopped
- Black pepper, to taste
- 1 cup nonfat yogurt
- 2 cups chicken stock
- 4 ¼ cups skinless white fish fillets, chopped into large chunks
- 1 ⅓ cups raw peeled king prawns
- 2 cups mussels, cleaned and debearded
- A small bunch flat-leaf parsley leaves, roughly chopped
- Crusty bread and almond butter, to serve (optional)

Directions:

1. Preheat the oil in a pan and sauté for onions for 5 minutes.
2. Add the pepper and garlic, and stir-cook for 2 minutes.
3. Pour in the stock and yogurt. Cook for 10 minutes.
4. Place the fish chunks in the pan and cook for 2 minutes.
5. Stir in the mussels and prawns. Cover the pan and cook for 3 minutes.
6. Garnish with parsley.
7. Serve.

Nutrition:

- Calories: 301
- Fats: 12.2 g
- Saturated Fat: 2.4 g
- Cholesterol: 110 mg
- Sodium: 276 mg
- Carbs: 5 g
- Fiber: 0.9 g
- Sugar: 1.4 g
- Protein: 28.8 g

4.   Fritto Misto With Gremolata

Preparation Time: 5 minutes
Cooking Time: 15 minutes
Servings: 4
Ingredients:
For the Gremolata:

- A small bunch flat-leaf parsley, finely chopped
- 1 lemon, zested
- ½ tsp. garlic, finely chopped

For the Fritto Misto:

- ⅓ cup (3-oz.) almond flour
- ¼ tsp. black pepper
- 2 ¼ cups cod fillet, bones removed and cut into bite-sized pieces
- 1 ⅓ cups mixed seafood
- 6 tbsp. olive oil
- Good-quality mayo, to serve

Directions:

1. Mix all the ingredients for the gremolata.
2. Combine the flour with the black pepper and seasoning in a bowl.
3. Dip the seafood in the flour mixture.
4. Preheat the oil in a frying pan and fry the coated seafood until golden brown.
5. Serve.

Nutrition:

- Calories: 310
- Fats: 2.4 g
- Saturated Fat: 0.1 g
- Cholesterol: 320 mg
- Sodium: 350 mg
- Carbs: 12.2 g
- Fiber: 0.7 g
- Sugar: 0.7 g
- Protein: 44.3 g

5.   Fritto Misto

Preparation Time: 5 minutes
Cooking Time: 10 minutes
Servings: 2
Ingredients:

- 1 cup Vegetable oil for deep frying
- 1 egg
- ½ pint whole milk
- 1 lb. mixed raw seafood, cut into pieces
- 1 zucchini, cut into batons
- ⅔ cup (4-oz.) almond flour
- 6 tbsp. corn flour
- ⅔ cup (4-oz.) semolina

Directions:

1. Preheat the oil to 320ºF in a deep pan.
2. Beat the milk with the egg white and seasonings.
3. Add the seafood and zucchini to the milk.
4. Combine corn flour, semolina, and flour in a bowl.
5. Dip the seafood and zucchini in the flour mixture, and shake off the excess.
6. Add the oil to a deep pan and heat to fry until golden.
7. Serve.

Nutrition:

- Calories: 372
- Fats: 1.1 g
- Saturated Fat: 3.8 g
- Cholesterol: 10 mg
- Sodium: 749 mg
- Carbs: 4.9 g
- Fiber: 0.2 g
- Sugar: 0.2 g
- Protein: 33.5 g

6.   Fish Soup

Preparation Time: 5 minutes
Cooking Time: 1 hour
Servings: 2
Ingredients:

- 2 tsp Olive oil
- 2 small onions, finely chopped
- 2 carrots, finely chopped
- 2 celery stalks, finely chopped
- 4 garlic cloves, finely chopped
- 1–2 sweet peppers, deseeded and finely chopped
- 2 ½ pints vegetable stock
- 4 cups fish stock
- 2 anchovy fillets in oil, drained
- Salt, pepper
- Pepper, pepper
- 2 ¼ cups (8-oz.) monkfish tail, all bones removed and flesh cut into cubes
- 2 ¼ cups (8-oz.) frozen seafood, defrosted and rinsed
- 2 handfuls small soup pasta
- A handful olives (black or green), pitted and finely chopped
- Fresh crusty bread, to serve

Directions:

1. Preheat the olive oil in the pan and sauté the onions, celery, peppers, and garlic until golden.
2. Stir in the stock, anchovy, and pepper.
3. Cover the lid and cook for 40 minutes.
4. Stir in the monkfish tail, pasta, and seafood.
5. Cover and cook for 20 minutes.
6. Serve with olives on top.
7. Enjoy.

Nutrition:

- Calories: 581
- Fats: 23 g
- Saturated Fat: 4 g
- Cholesterol: 49 mg
- Sodium: 257 mg
- Carbs: 3.6 g
- Fiber: 10 g
- Sugar: 0.5 g
- Protein: 58 g

7.   Chicken Chasseur

Preparation Time: 5 minutes
Cooking Time: 30 minutes
Servings: 4
Ingredients:

- 4 chicken legs
- 1 tbsp. olive oil
- 1 onion, finely sliced
- 2 garlic cloves, finely sliced
- 2 ¼ cups (8-oz.) chestnut mushrooms, cut into 4 if small and 6 if large
- 3 ½ cups chicken stock
- 1 bay leaf
- 1 thyme sprig
- 1 cup nonfat yogurt
- 1 red bell pepper, chopped
- A small handful of tarragon, chopped
- Mashed potatoes, to serve

Directions:

1. Sear the chicken legs in some oil until golden brown.
2. Remove the chicken and sauté onion until soft.
3. Add mushrooms and garlic until golden.
4. Stir in nonfat yogurt, bay leaf, thyme, red bell pepper, and chicken stock.
5. Boil the mixture and then reduce it to a simmer. Add the chicken legs.
6. Cook for 30 minutes and add the tarragon.
7. Serve.

Nutrition:

- Calories: 529
- Fats: 17 g
- Saturated Fat: 3 g
- Cholesterol: 65 mg
- Sodium: 391 mg
- Carbs: 55 g
- Fiber: 6 g
- Sugar: 8 g
- Protein: 41 g

8.   Smoky Chicken Traybake

Preparation Time: 10 minutes
Cooking Time: 45 minutes
Servings: 4
Ingredients:

- 1 (2-lb.) pack chicken thighs and drumsticks
- Olive oil, for greasing
- 1 red bell pepper, deseeded and roughly chopped
- 2 yellow bell peppers, deseeded and roughly chopped
- 2 red onions, peeled and sliced into wedges
- ½ cups barbecue sauce
- 7 ¼ cups sweet potatoes, scrubbed and cut into wedges
- ⅔ cup sour cream
- Coriander leaves, to garnish
- Guacamole, to serve

Directions:

1. Set the oven to 400°F. Score the skin of the thighs.
2. Place them with the peppers and the red onion in the roasting pan.
3. Mix all the remaining ingredients.
4. Top the chicken and vegetables with this paste.
5. Roast the chicken for 15 minutes and then add sweet potato.
6. Turn all the drumsticks and bake for 30 minutes.
7. Serve.

Nutrition:

- Calories: 284
- Fats: 25 g
- Saturated Fat: 1 g
- Cholesterol: 49 mg
- Sodium: 460 mg
- Carbs: 35 g
- Fiber: 2 g
- Sugar: 6 g
- Protein: 26 g

9.   Chicken and Orzo Bake

Preparation Time: 5 minutes
Cooking Time: 40 minutes
Servings: 4
Ingredients:

- ½ tbsp. olive oil
- 4 (2 1/5-lb.) pack bone-in chicken thighs
- 2 onions, finely chopped
- 2 celery sticks, finely chopped
- 1 carrot, peeled and finely chopped
- 1 garlic clove, finely chopped
- 1 tsp. fennel seeds
- 2 cups orzo
- 1 chicken stock cube, made up with 2 cups hot water
- 2 cups frozen broccoli florets
- A handful fresh dill, chopped
- 1 lemon, cut into wedges to serve
- Pepper, to taste

Directions:

1. Preheat the oil in a deep cooking pan.
2. Season the chicken and cook for 5 minutes per side.
3. Remove the chicken from the cooking pan and keep it aside.
4. Drain the excess fat and keep it aside.
5. Add the onion, carrot, celery, garlic, and fennel seeds to the pan.
6. Stir-cook for 10 minutes and then add stock and orzo.
7. Return the chicken to the pan.
8. Boil the mixture and cook on simmer for 5 minutes.
9. Add the broccoli and cook for 20 minutes.
10. Garnish with dill and pepper.
11. Serve.

Nutrition:

- Calories: 152
- Fats: 4 g
- Saturated Fat: 2 g
- Cholesterol: 65 mg
- Sodium: 220 mg
- Carbs: 1 tsp.
- Fiber: 0 g
- Sugar: 1 g
- Protein: 26 g

10.   One-Pot Roast

Preparation Time: 10 minutes
Cooking Time: 50 minutes
Servings: 8
Ingredients:

- 8 chicken thighs
- 1 ½ lb. sweet potato, cut into chunks
- 2 cups (7-oz.) chorizo sausage, sliced
- 1 bulb garlic, broken into cloves
- 2 tbsp. grapeseed oil
- ⅓ cup chicken stock
- 1 lemon, halved
- 2 zucchinis, cut into thick batons
- 1 red chili, deseeded and sliced
- 2 1/6 cup (8-oz.) baby spinach
- 2 tbsp. parsley, chopped
- A pinch salt
- A pinch black pepper

Directions:

1. Set the oven to 400°F.
2. Place the chicken with the sweet potato in a roasting pan.
3. Top the chicken with garlic, grapeseed oil, stock, and lemon juice.
4. Bake for 50 minutes. Add the zucchini, chili, and chorizo after 30 minutes of baking.
5. Garnish with the parsley and spinach.
6. Serve.

Nutrition:

- Calories: 188
- Fats: 8 g
- Saturated Fat: 1 g
- Cholesterol: 0 mg
- Sodium: 339 mg
- Carbs: 8 g
- Fiber: 1 g
- Sugar: 2 g
- Protein: 13 g

11.　Beef Curry

Preparation Time: 10 minutes
Cooking Time: 22 minutes
Servings: 4
Ingredients:

- 14 oz. beef rump, sliced thinly
- ¼ cup sunflower oil
- 1 cup brown rice
- 4 ¼ cups boiling water
- 1 tbsp. fresh ginger, minced
- A few slices of fresh ginger
- 2 garlic cloves, minced
- 1 tsp. ground cumin
- 1 tsp. ground coriander
- 1 tsp. turmeric
- 1 tsp. ground black pepper
- ½ tsp. chili powder
- ½ tsp. ground ginger
- ½ cup frozen peas
- Coriander sprigs, to garnish
- Salt, to taste

Directions:

1. Boil the rice in salted water and cook for 12 minutes. Drain and keep aside.
2. Preheat the sunflower oil in the pan, and sear the beef until brown.
3. Remove the beef to the plate lined with a paper towel.
4. Add the ginger and garlic, and sauté for few minutes.
5. Stir in the spices and water.
6. Cook for 10 minutes, then add peas.
7. Adjust the seasoning, and garnish with coriander.
8. Serve.

Nutrition:

- Calories: 301
- Fats: 15.8 g
- Saturated Fat: 2.7 g
- Cholesterol: 75 mg
- Sodium: 1189 mg
- Carbs: 11.7 g
- Fiber: 0.3 g
- Sugar: 0.1 g
- Protein: 28.2 g

12.　Beef Schnitzel

Preparation Time: 10 minutes
Cooking Time: 30 minutes
Servings: 6
Ingredients:

- 4 tbsp. almond flour
- 1 large egg, beaten
- 1 ¼ cup (5-oz.) breadcrumbs
- 2 (3 1/6) cups beef medallion steaks
- 2 tbsp. olive oil
- 1 lemon, cut into wedges to serve

For the slaw:

- 2 raw beetroots, peeled and grated
- 1 large carrot, peeled and grated
- ½ red onion, peeled and finely sliced
- 2 stalks celery, finely sliced
- ½ pack dill, leaves chopped
- 1 lemon, zested and juiced
- 1 tbsp. extra-virgin olive oil

Directions:

1. Combine everything for the slaw in a bowl. Adjust the seasoning with salt.
2. Mix the flour with the lemon zest and salt.
3. Beat the egg white in a bowl, and spread breadcrumbs in a shallow bowl.
4. Place each beef medallion in between 2 sheets of parchment paper.
5. Pound the meat using a rolling pin to reduce the thickness.
6. First, dip the meat into the flour mixture; then add the egg, and then breadcrumbs.
7. Preheat the oil in a frying pan, and cook the coated meat for 2 minutes per side.
8. Serve with slaw.

Nutrition:

- Calories: 308
- Fats: 20.5 g
- Saturated Fat: 3 g
- Cholesterol: 0 mg
- Sodium: 688 mg
- Carbs: 10.3 g
- Sugar: 1.4 g
- Fiber: 4.3 g
- Protein: 49 g

13. Beef Massaman Curry

Preparation Time: 10 minutes
Cooking Time: 31 minutes
Servings: 6
Ingredients:
- 1 ½ tbsp. vegetable oil
- 2 onions, chopped
- 2 ¼ cups Thai jasmine rice
- 2 cups Thai massaman paste
- 3 cups potatoes, cut into 2 cm-thick slices
- 5 ¼ cups cooked roast beef, cut into chunks
- 1 ⅓ cups pack baby corn and snap peas
- Water, as needed
- 2 tbsp Star anise

Directions:
1. Preheat the oil in a deep-frying pan, and sauté the onions for 10 minutes on low heat.
2. Boil the rice in salted water for 10 minutes, and then drain and keep them aside.
3. Add the massaman paste and cook for 1 minute.
4. Put in the sliced potato, coconut milk, and star anise.
5. Cook this mixture for 15 minutes.
6. Add snap peas, a splash of water, corn, and beef.
7. Cook for 5 minutes, then serve.

Nutrition:
- Calories: 231
- Fats: 20.1 g
- Saturated Fat: 2.4 g
- Cholesterol: 110 mg
- Sodium: 941 mg
- Carbs: 20.1 g
- Fiber: 0.9 g
- Sugar: 1.4 g
- Protein: 14.6 g

14. Barbecued Rump of Beef in Dijon

Preparation Time: 10 minutes
Cooking Time: 1 hour and 45 minutes
Servings: 4
Ingredients:
- 2 lb. beef top rump joint
- 2 tbsp. fresh tarragon, roughly chopped
- 2 tsp. black pepper
- 1 tbsp. Dijon mustard
- 2 tbsp. olive oil

Directions:
1. Keep the meat in a shallow dish and toss with tarragon, mustard, oil, and pepper to season.
2. Marinate the meat in the refrigerator for 1 ½ hours.
3. Preheat the grill and grill for 15 minutes.
4. Carve and serve.

Nutrition:
- Calories: 280
- Fats: 3.5 g
- Saturated Fat: 0.1 g
- Cholesterol: 320 mg
- Sodium: 350 mg
- Carbs: 7.6 g
- Fiber: 0.7 g
- Sugar: 0.7 g
- Protein: 11.2 g

15.   Roast Rib of Beef

Preparation Time: 10 minutes
Cooking Time: 45 minutes
Servings: 6
Ingredients:

- 2 Knorr® Beef Stock Cubes
- 1 tbsp. olive oil
- 3 lb. rib of beef
- 5 small leeks
- 6 parsnips, peeled and halved
- 6 carrots, peeled and halved
- 4 shallots, peeled and halved
- Celery sticks, cut into large chunks, for serving
- Fresh sage leaves, for serving

Directions:

1. Set the oven to 400°F.
2. Mix 1 Knorr beef cube with 1 tablespoon of oil and rub this paste onto the beef.
3. Sear the beef in a greased pan until brown, then transfer them to a roasting pan.
4. Sauté the leeks in the same pan until golden, and place them around the beef.
5. Now sauté carrots and parsnips in the pan and also transfer them to the roasting pan.
6. Top the beef with sage, celery, and shallots.
7. Bake for 45 minutes.
8. Serve.

Nutrition:

- Calories: 472
- Fats: 11.1 g
- Saturated Fat: 5.8 g
- Cholesterol: 610 mg
- Sodium: 749 mg
- Carbs: 19.9 g
- Fiber: 0.2 g
- Sugar: 0.2 g
- Protein: 13.5 g

16.   Beef Wellington with Stilton

Preparation Time: 5 minutes
Cooking Time: 55 minutes
Servings: 4
Ingredients:

- 2 tbsp. olive oil
- 2 tbsp. pine nuts
- 1 garlic clove, crushed
- 4 tbsp. horseradish sauce
- ¼ cup (2-oz.) mature stilton, crumbled
- 1 oz. fresh white breadcrumbs
- 1 (1 ½-lb.) beef fillet piece
- 3 ⅓ cups (13-oz.) ready-rolled puff pastry
- Beaten egg, to glaze

Directions:

1. Preheat 1 tablespoon of oil in a frying pan and sauté the pine nuts for 1 minute.
2. Toss in the garlic and set the mixture aside to cool.
3. Combine the stilton, horseradish, breadcrumbs, black pepper, and pine nuts mixture.
4. Heat more oil in a pan and sear beef fillet for 3 minutes per side, or until brown.
5. Adjust the oven to 400°F.
6. Top the beef with the horseradish mixture.
7. Spread the pastry sheet and top the beef pan with it.
8. Brush the pastry with the beaten egg white.
9. Seal the edges and bake for 40 minutes.
10. Serve.

Nutrition:

- Calories: 327
- Fats: 3.5 g
- Saturated Fat: 0.5 g
- Cholesterol: 162 mg
- Sodium: 142 mg
- Carbs: 33.6 g
- Fiber: 0.4 g
- Sugar: 0.5 g
- Protein: 24.5 g

17.   Marinated Lamb Steaks

Preparation Time: 10 minutes
Cooking Time: 30 minutes
Servings: 6
Ingredients:

- 6 lamb leg steaks
- ½ cup dark coconut aminos
- 1 tbsp. curry powder
- 1 tsp. ground ginger
- 1 tbsp. nonfat yogurt
- 1 tbsp. olive oil
- Salt, to taste
- Pepper, to taste
- 2 cups fresh potatoes
- ⅔ cup pot natural yogurt
- A bunch mint
- A bunch spring onions
- Salted water, as needed

Directions:

1. Combine everything for the marinade and rub it over the lamb steaks.
2. Let it marinate for 1 hour at room temperature.
3. Meanwhile, boil the potatoes in the salted water, drain them, and let them cool down.
4. Mix the yogurt with spring onion and mint.
5. Toss in the potatoes and seasonings.
6. Preheat the grill and grill the lamb steaks for 3 minutes per side.
7. Serve with the potato mixture.

Nutrition:

- Calories: 413
- Fats: 7.5 g
- Saturated Fat: 1.1 g
- Cholesterol: 20 mg
- Sodium: 97 mg
- Carbs: 41.4 g
- Fiber: 0 g
- Sugar: 0 g
- Protein: 21.1 g

18.   Lamb Kofta Curry

Preparation Time: 10 minutes
Cooking Time: 50 minutes
Servings: 4
Ingredients:

- 6 lamb leg steaks
- ½ cup dark coconut aminos
- 1 tbsp. curry powder
- 1 tsp. ground ginger
- 1 tbsp. nonfat yogurt
- 1 tbsp. olive oil
- Salt, to taste
- Pepper, to taste
- 2 cups fresh potatoes
- ⅔ cup pot natural yogurt
- A bunch mint
- A bunch spring onions

Directions:

1. Combine everything for the marinade and rub it over the lamb steaks.
2. Let it marinate for 1 hour at room temperature.
3. Meanwhile, boil the potatoes in the salted water, drain them, and let them cool down.
4. Mix the yogurt with the spring onion and mint.
5. Toss in the potatoes and seasonings.
6. Preheat the grill and grill the lamb steaks for 3 minutes per side.
7. Serve with the potato mixture.

Nutrition:

- Calories: 413
- Fats: 7.5 g
- Saturated Fat: 1.1 g
- Cholesterol: 20 mg
- Sodium: 97 mg
- Carbs: 41.4 g
- Fiber: 0 g
- Sugar: 0 g
- Protein: 21.1 g

19. Mediterranean Lamb Stew with Olives

Preparation Time: 1–5 minutes
Cooking Time: 1 hour and 20 minutes
Servings: 4
Ingredients:

- ½ lb. lamb leg steaks, cut into 1-inch chunks
- 2 tsp. cold-pressed rapeseed oil
- 2 medium onions, 1 thinly sliced, 1 cut into 5 wedges
- 2 garlic cloves, peeled and finely sliced
- ¼ cup dried split red lentils, rinsed
- ¾ cup water
- 2 tbsp Thyme
- 2 Orange peel

Directions:

1. Add the oil to a suitable pan and heat it.
2. Sear the lamb for 10 minutes, or until brown. Transfer it to a plate lined with pepper.
3. Heat more oil and sauté the onions for 5 minutes.
4. Stir in the garlic and cook for 30 seconds.
5. Return the lamb to the pan.
6. Add the thyme, ¾ cup water, and orange peel.
7. Let it cook on a low simmer for 1 hour.
8. Stir in the olives. Cook for 20 minutes, then serve.

Nutrition:

- Calories: 201
- Fats: 5.5 g
- Saturated Fat: 2.1 g
- Cholesterol: 10 mg
- Sodium: 597 mg
- Carbs: 2.4 g
- Fiber: 0 g
- Sugar: 0 g
- Protein: 3.1 g

20. Herb and Spiced Lamb

Preparation Time: 10 minutes
Cooking Time: 20 minutes
Servings: 4
Ingredients:

- 14 oz. lamb neck fillet, trimmed of sinew and excess fat
- ½ tbsp. cumin
- ½ tbsp. ground coriander
- 1 tbsp. coriander seeds, toasted and bashed
- 2 tbsp. olive oil, plus a drizzle
- A bunch mint, leaves picked
- A bunch dill, chopped
- A bunch coriander, leaves picked
- 2 cups feta
- 1 pomegranate, seeds only
- 1 lemon, juiced

Directions:

1. Set the oven to 400°F.
2. Season the lamb with the spices.
3. Heat the oil in a suitable frying pan and sear the lamb for 3 minutes per side.
4. Place it on a baking sheet and roast it for 10 minutes in the oven.
5. Top the lamb with the remaining ingredients and serve.

Nutrition:

- Calories: 413
- Fats: 8.5 g
- Saturated Fat: 3.1 g
- Cholesterol: 120 mg
- Sodium: 497 mg
- Carbs: 21.4 g
- Fiber: 0.6 g
- Sugar: 0.1 g
- Protein: 14.1 g

21.   Simple Vegetable Broth

Preparation Time: 10 minutes
Cooking Time: 2 hours
Servings: 8
Ingredients:

- 2 carrots, peeled and roughly chopped
- 1 leek, green part only, roughly chopped and washed (see headnote)
- 1 celery stalk, roughly chopped
- 1 fennel bulb, roughly chopped
- 9 cups water

Directions:

1. In a large pot, combine all the ingredients.
2. Bring to a simmer over medium-high heat, then lower the heat to low and simmer for 2 hours.
3. Strain the vegetables from the broth, and store the broth until you're ready to use it.

Nutrition:

- Calories: 10
- Protein: 0 g
- Fats: 0 g
- Saturated Fat: 0 g
- Carbs: 3 g
- Fiber: 0 g
- Sodium: 20 mg

22.   Cooling Cucumber Soup

Preparation Time: 10 minutes
Cooking Time: 0 minutes
Servings: 4
Ingredients:

- 4 medium cucumbers, roughly chopped
- ½ avocado, peeled, pitted, and roughly chopped
- 1 cup baby spinach, finely chopped
- ¼ cup fresh cilantro, chopped
- 1 tsp. ginger root, grated
- 1 lime, zested
- ½ tsp. sea salt
- 3 cups simple vegetable broth
- ½ cup lactose-free plain nonfat yogurt
- 2 tbsp. extra-virgin olive oil
- Baby spinach leaves (optional, for garnish)

Directions:

1. In a blender or food processor, combine the cucumbers, avocado, spinach, cilantro, ginger, lime zest, salt, vegetable broth, yogurt, and olive oil. Blend until smooth.
2. Chill for at least 2 hours.
3. Garnish with spinach leaves just before serving (if using).

Nutrition:

- Calories: 183
- Protein: 4 g
- Fats: 13 g
- Saturated Fat: 3 g
- Carbs: 16 g
- Fiber: 4 g
- Sodium: 265 mg

23. Miso Soup with Tofu and Greens

Preparation Time: 10 minutes
Cooking Time: 3 minutes
Servings: 4
Ingredients:

- 1 tbsp. olive oil
- 1 leek, green part only, chopped and washed (see headnote)
- 3 oz. extra-firm tofu, cut into ¼-inch cubes
- 7 cups simple vegetable broth, divided
- 3 cups baby spinach
- 2 tbsp. miso paste

Directions:

1. In a large nonstick pot, heat the olive oil over medium-high heat until it shimmers.
2. Add the leek and tofu and cook, stirring occasionally, until the leek is soft, about 5 minutes.
3. Add 6 cups of broth. Bring to a simmer and lower the heat to medium.
4. Add the spinach. Cook for 3 minutes.
5. In a small bowl, whisk together the remaining 1 cup of broth and the miso paste. Stir into the hot soup. Cook for 30 seconds more, stirring.

Nutrition:

- Calories: 117
- Protein: 8 g
- Fats: 6 g
- Saturated Fat: 1 g
- Carbs: 12 g
- Fiber: 2 g
- Sodium: 1342 mg

24. Italian Vegetable Soup

Preparation Time: 10 minutes
Cooking Time: 17 minutes
Servings: 4
Ingredients:

- 1 tbsp. olive oil
- 1 leek, green part only, chopped and washed (see headnote, here)
- 1 carrot, peeled and chopped
- 1 zucchini, chopped
- 1 cup green beans, trimmed and chopped
- 1 cup canned kidney beans
- 1 tbsp. dried Italian seasoning
- ½ tsp. sea salt
- 7 cups simple vegetable broth
- 2 tbsp. fresh basil, chopped

Directions:

1. In a large nonstick pot, heat the olive oil over medium-high heat until it shimmers.
2. Add the leek, carrot, and zucchini and cook, stirring occasionally, until the leek is soft, about 5 minutes.
3. Add the green beans, kidney beans, Italian seasoning, salt, and vegetable broth. Bring to a simmer, then lower the heat to medium. Simmer, stirring occasionally, until the green beans are tender, about 5 to 7 minutes.
4. Stir in the basil just before serving.

Nutrition:

- Calories: 120
- Protein: 5 g
- Fats: 4 g
- Saturated Fat: <1 g
- Carbs: 18 g
- Fiber: 6 g
- Sodium: 445 mg

25. Creamy Pumpkin Soup

Preparation Time: 10 minutes
Cooking Time: 12 minutes
Servings: 4
Ingredients:

- 1 tbsp. olive oil
- 1 leek, green part only, finely chopped and washed (see headnote)
- 1 cup canned pure pumpkin (not pumpkin pie filling)
- 3 cups simple vegetable broth
- 1 tsp. dried sage
- ½ tsp. sea salt
- ½ cup light coconut milk
- 1 tsp. cornstarch

Directions:

1. In a large saucepan, heat the olive oil over medium-high heat until it shimmers.
2. Add the leek and cook, stirring, until soft, about 5 minutes.
3. Add the pumpkin, vegetable broth, sage, and salt. Bring to a simmer and cook for 5 minutes.
4. In a small bowl, whisk together the coconut milk and cornstarch.
5. Remove the pan from the heat and carefully pour the soup into a blender or food processor, along with the coconut milk and cornstarch. Allow the steam to escape through the hole in the blender lid or the food processor feed tube as you blend, to avoid a buildup of pressure. Blend until smooth.
6. Return the soup to the pot and warm over medium heat for 2 minutes, or until thick.

Nutrition:

- Calories: 92
- Protein: 2 g
- Fats: 5 g
- Saturated Fat: 2 g
- Carbs: 10 g
- Fiber: 2 g
- Sodium: 245 mg

26. Cream of Broccoli Soup

Preparation Time: 10 minutes
Cooking Time: 15 minutes
Servings: 4
Ingredients:

- 1 tbsp. olive oil
- 1 leek, green part only, washed and finely chopped
- 3 cups broccoli florets
- 6 cups simple vegetable broth
- ½ tsp. sea salt
- 1 cup lactose-free nonfat milk
- 1 tbsp. cornstarch
- ¼ cup lactose-free nonfat plain yogurt, for garnish (optional)
- ½ cup baby kale, for garnish (optional)
- ¼ cup microgreens, for garnish (optional)

Directions:

1. In a large pot, heat the olive oil over medium-high heat until it shimmers.
2. Add the leek and broccoli and cook, stirring, until the leek is soft, about 5 minutes.
3. Add the vegetable broth and salt. Bring to a simmer. Lower the heat to medium and simmer, stirring occasionally, until the broccoli is soft, about 5 minutes.
4. In a small bowl, whisk together the milk and cornstarch. Stir the mixture into the soup. Cook for a few minutes more, stirring, until the soup thickens slightly.
5. Thin the yogurt (if using) with a little water. Drizzle it on the soup as a garnish.
6. Garnish with the kale and microgreens (if using).

Nutrition:

- Calories: 127
- Protein: 6 g
- Fats: 4 g
- Saturated Fat: <1 g
- Carbs: 19 g
- Fiber: 4 g
- Sodium: 401 mg

27. Sweet Potato and Corn Stew

Preparation Time: 10 minutes
Cooking Time: 15 minutes
Servings: 2
Ingredients:

- 1 tbsp. olive oil
- 1 leek, green part only, finely chopped and washed
- 2 cups spinach
- 1 medium sweet potato, peeled and cut into ½-inch cubes (1 cup or less)
- ½ cup canned or frozen corn
- 3 cups simple vegetable broth
- 2 tsp. cornstarch
- 1 tsp. dried cumin
- ½ tsp. sea salt
- 1 cup lactose-free nonfat plain yogurt
- ¼ cup fresh cilantro, chopped
- ½ tsp. lime zest, grated

Directions:

1. In a large saucepan, heat the olive oil over medium-high heat until it shimmers.
2. Add the leek and cook, stirring occasionally, until soft, about 5 minutes.
3. Add the spinach, sweet potato, and corn.
4. In a bowl, whisk together the vegetable broth, cornstarch, cumin, and salt. Add to the pan and bring to a simmer.
5. Lower the heat to medium. Cook, stirring occasionally, until the sweet potato is soft, about 10 minutes.
6. Stir in the yogurt, cilantro, and lime zest just before serving.

Nutrition:

- Calories: 248
- Protein: 8 g
- Fats: 8 g
- Saturated Fat: 2 g
- Carbs: 39 g
- Fiber: 5 g
- Sodium: 613 mg

28. Broccoli and Cheese Baked Potato

Preparation Time: 10 minutes
Cooking Time: 1 hour and 30 minutes
Servings: 2
Ingredients:

- 2 small russet potatoes
- 1 cup broccoli florets
- ½ tsp. sea salt
- ½ cup Cheddar cheese, grated

Directions:

1. Preheat the oven to 350°F. Pierce the potatoes several times with a fork.
2. Bake the potatoes on a rimmed baking sheet for 1 hour. Add the broccoli to the pan in a single layer. Continue to roast for 30 minutes, or until the potatoes are soft and the broccoli is tender.
3. Split the potatoes. Season with the salt and top with the broccoli and Cheddar. (Melt the cheese in the microwave for about 45 seconds, if desired.)

Nutrition:

- Calories: 247
- Protein: 11 g
- Fats: 10 g
- Saturated Fat: 6 g
- Carbs: 30 g
- Fiber: 5 g
- Sodium: 669 mg

29.   Lentil Tacos

Preparation Time: 10 minutes
Cooking Time: 10 minutes
Servings: 4
Ingredients:

- 4 small corn tortillas
- 1 tbsp. olive oil
- 1 leek, green part only, chopped and washed
- 2 cups canned lentils
- ¼ cup simple vegetable broth
- 1 tsp. ground cumin
- ½ tsp. ground coriander
- ½ tsp. sea salt
- ¼ avocado, chopped
- ¼ cup fresh cilantro, chopped

Directions:

1. Preheat the oven to 350°F. Wrap the tortillas in aluminum foil and put them in the oven to warm for 15 minutes.
2. Meanwhile, in a large saucepan, heat the olive oil over medium-high heat until it shimmers. Add the leek and cook until soft, about 5 minutes.
3. Add the lentils, vegetable broth, cumin, coriander, and salt. Bring to a simmer and then lower the heat to medium. Simmer, stirring occasionally, for 5 minutes.
4. To serve, spoon the lentils onto the tortillas, and top with the avocado and cilantro.

Nutrition:

- Calories: 256
- Protein: 9 g
- Fats: 8 g
- Saturated Fat: 1 g
- Carbs: 37 g
- Fiber: 6 g
- Sodium: 366 mg

30.   Pasta with Walnut Pesto

Preparation Time: 0 minutes
Cooking Time: 0 minutes
Servings: 2
Ingredients:

- ¼ cup tightly packed fresh basil leaves
- ¼ cup walnuts
- ¼ cup grated Parmesan cheese
- 1 tbsp. olive oil
- 1 tsp. grated lemon zest
- ½ tsp. sea salt
- 1 cup dry gluten-free penne, cooked according to package instructions and drained

Directions:

1. In a blender or food processor, combine the basil, walnuts, Parmesan, olive oil, lemon zest, and salt.
2. Pulse 15 to 20 times, or until well chopped.
3. Toss the pesto with the hot cooked pasta.

Nutrition:

- Calories: 293
- Protein: 9 g
- Fats: 13 g
- Saturated Fat: 3 g
- Carbs: 38 g
- Fiber: 2 g
- Sodium: 598 mg

31. Zucchini and Carrot Frittata

Preparation Time: 10 minutes
Cooking Time: 13 minutes
Servings: 4
Ingredients:

- 1 tbsp. olive oil
- 1 carrot, peeled and chopped
- 1 zucchini, grated
- 4 large eggs
- 1 tbsp. fresh thyme, chopped
- ¼ tsp. sea salt

Directions:

1. Preheat the broiler on high.
2. In a large, oven-safe nonstick skillet, heat the olive oil over medium-high heat until it shimmers.
3. Add the carrot and cook, stirring occasionally, until it begins to soften, about 3 minutes.
4. Add the zucchini and cook for 2 minutes.
5. In a medium bowl, whisk the eggs with the thyme and salt.
6. Spread out the vegetables evenly in the bottom of the skillet.
7. Carefully pour the eggs over the top. Lower the heat to medium.
8. Cook until the eggs begin to set around the edges, about 2 minutes. Using a spatula, carefully pull the set eggs away from the sides of the skillet. Tilt the skillet to distribute the uncooked egg into the space you've made. Cook until the eggs set around the edges again, about 2 to 3 minutes more.
9. Transfer the skillet to the broiler. Broil until set on top, about 2 to 3 minutes.
10. Cut it into wedges to serve.

Nutrition:

- Calories: 116
- Protein: 7 g
- Fats: 9 g
- Saturated Fat: 2 g
- Carbs: 4 g
- Fiber: 1 g
- Sodium: 195 mg

32. Zucchini Ribbons with Parmesan Cream Sauce

Preparation Time: 10 minutes
Cooking Time: 5 minutes
Servings: 2
Ingredients:

- 1 tbsp. olive oil
- 3 small zucchinis, cut into ribbons with a vegetable peeler
- ½ tsp. sea salt
- ½ cup lactose-free nonfat milk
- ¼ cup Parmesan cheese, grated

Directions:

1. In a large, nonstick skillet, heat the olive oil over medium-high heat until it shimmers.
2. Add the zucchini and salt and cook, stirring occasionally, until tender, about 4 minutes.
3. While the zucchini is being cooked, heat the milk in a small saucepan over medium heat. When it simmers, whisk in the Parmesan.
4. Cook the milk mixture, stirring, until smooth. Toss with the cooked zucchini.

Nutrition:

- Calories: 177
- Protein: 11 g
- Fats: 11 g
- Saturated Fat: 3 g
- Carbs: 12 g
- Fiber: 2 g
- Sodium: 681 mg

33. Asian Veggie and Tofu Stir-Fry

Preparation Time: 10 minutes
Cooking Time: 10 minutes
Servings: 2
Ingredients:

- ¼ cup simple vegetable broth
- 1 tsp. miso paste
- ½ tsp. fresh ginger, grated
- ½ tsp. orange zest, grated
- ½ tsp. sea salt
- 1 tbsp. olive oil
- 6 oz. extra-firm tofu, cut into ½-inch cubes
- 1 leek, green part only, chopped and washed (see headnote)
- 2 carrots, peeled and chopped
- 2 cups bok choy, chopped

Directions:

1. In a small bowl, whisk together the broth, miso, ginger, orange zest, and salt. Set aside.
2. In a large, nonstick skillet, heat the olive oil over medium-high heat until it shimmers.
3. Add the tofu, leek, carrots, and bok choy. Cook, stirring occasionally, until the veggies begin to brown, about 5 to 7 minutes.
4. Add the reserved sauce and bring to a simmer. Cook, stirring, until the sauce thickens, about 3 to 4 minutes more.

Nutrition:

- Calories: 206
- Protein: 11 g
- Fats: 12 g
- Saturated Fat: 2 g
- Carbs: 17 g
- Fiber: 4 g
- Sodium: 681 mg

34. Soba Noodles with Peanut Butter Sauce

Preparation Time: 10 minutes
Cooking Time: 10 minutes
Servings: 2
Ingredients:

- ¼ cup peanut butter
- ¼ cup light coconut milk
- 1 tsp. miso paste
- 1 tsp. fresh ginger, grated
- 2 tbsp. fresh cilantro, chopped
- Water or simple vegetable broth (optional)
- 2 oz. soba (buckwheat) noodles, cooked according to package instructions and drained

Directions:

1. In a small saucepan, combine the peanut butter, coconut milk, miso, ginger, and cilantro.
2. Cook over medium-high heat, stirring, until melted and blended. Thin with a little water or broth if needed.
3. Toss with the hot noodles.

Nutrition:

- Calories: 311
- Protein: 13 g
- Fats: 19 g
- Saturated Fat: 5 g
- Carbs: 27 g
- Fiber: 3 g
- Sodium: 263 mg

35. Brown Rice and Peanut Lettuce Wraps

Preparation Time: 10 minutes
Cooking Time: 9 minutes
Servings: 2
Ingredients:

- 1 tbsp. olive oil
- 1 leek, green part only, finely chopped and washed (see headnote)
- 3 oz. extra-firm tofu, cut into ¼-inch cubes
- 1 ½ cups cooked brown rice
- 2 tbsp. crunchy peanut butter
- 1 tbsp. fresh ginger, grated
- ¼ cup simple vegetable broth
- ½ tsp. sea salt
- 2 tbsp. fresh cilantro, chopped
- 4 large lettuce leaves

Directions:

1. In a nonstick skillet, heat the olive oil over medium-high heat until it shimmers. Add the leek and tofu and cook, stirring, until the leek is soft, about 5 minutes.
2. Add the rice, peanut butter, ginger, broth, and salt. Cook, stirring constantly, until well blended and hot, about 4 minutes.
3. Stir in the cilantro.
4. Spoon the rice mixture into the lettuce leaves, roll them up, and serve.

Nutrition:

- Calories: 445
- Protein: 14 g
- Fats: 27 g
- Saturated Fat: 4 g
- Carbs: 38 g
- Fiber: 4 g
- Sodium: 603 mg

36. Vegetable and Tofu Fried Rice

Preparation Time: 10 minutes
Cooking Time: 9 minutes
Servings: 4
Ingredients:

- 1 tbsp. olive oil
- 1 leek, green part only, washed and finely chopped
- 1 carrot, peeled and chopped
- ½ cup broccoli florets
- 3 oz. extra-firm tofu, cut into ¼-inch pieces
- 1 tbsp. fresh ginger, grated
- 3 cups cooked brown rice
- ¼ cup simple vegetable broth
- 1 tsp. miso paste

Directions:

1. In a nonstick skillet, heat the olive oil over medium-high heat until it shimmers. Add the leek, carrot, broccoli, tofu, and ginger. Then cook, stirring, until the veggies are soft, about 5 minutes.
2. Add the rice.
3. In a small bowl, whisk together the broth and miso. Add the mixture to the rice.
4. Stir-cook until warmed through, about 3 to 4 minutes more.

Nutrition:

- Calories: 189
- Protein: 5 g
- Fats: 6 g
- Saturated Fat: 1 g
- Carbs: 30 g
- Fiber: 2 g
- Sodium: 77 mg

37.   Butternut Risotto

Preparation Time: 5 minutes
Cooking Time: 16 minutes
Servings: 2
Ingredients:

- 2 cups simple vegetable broth
- 1 tbsp. olive oil
- 1 cup butternut squash, cubed
- ½ cup Arborio rice
- 1 tsp. dried thyme
- ½ tsp. sea salt
- ¼ cup Parmesan cheese, grated

Directions:

1. In a medium saucepan, heat the broth over medium-low heat and keep warm.
2. In a large saucepan, heat the olive oil over medium-high heat until it shimmers. Add the squash and cook, stirring until it starts to brown, about 4 minutes.
3. Add the rice and thyme. Stir-cook for 1 minute.
4. One ladleful at a time, add the hot broth, stirring constantly. As the rice starts to look dry, ladle in more broth until the rice is tender. This process will take about 15 minutes in total.
5. Turn off the heat and stir in the salt and Parmesan.

Nutrition:

- Calories: 196
- Protein: 7 g
- Fats: 10 g
- Saturated Fat: 3 g
- Carbs: 22 g
- Fiber: 3 g
- Sodium: 622 mg

38.   Brown Rice and Tofu with Kale

Preparation Time: 10 minutes
Cooking Time: 7 minutes
Servings: 2
Ingredients:

- 1 tbsp. olive oil
- ½ leek, green part only, chopped and washed
- 1 cup kale, stemmed and chopped
- 1 carrot, peeled and chopped
- 1 fennel bulb, cored and chopped
- 1 tsp. dried oregano
- 1 cup simple vegetable broth
- 1 ½ cups cooked brown rice
- ½ tsp. sea salt
- ½ tsp. orange zest, grated

Directions:

1. In a large saucepan, heat the olive oil over medium-high heat until it shimmers. Add the leek, kale, carrot, fennel, and oregano. Cook, stirring occasionally, until the vegetables are soft, about 5 minutes.
2. Add the broth, rice, and salt. Stir-cook for 2 minutes, or until the broth reduces.
3. Stir in the orange zest.

Nutrition:

- Calories: 254
- Protein: 5 g
- Fats: 8 g
- Saturated Fat: 1 g
- Carbs: 43 g
- Fiber: 6 g
- Sodium: 582 mg

39. Seasoned Tofu with Chimichurri

Preparation Time: 10 minutes
Cooking Time: 10 minutes
Servings: 2
Ingredients:

- ½ tsp. dried oregano
- ½ tsp. ground cumin
- ½ tsp. ground coriander
- ½ tsp. sea salt
- 6 oz. extra-firm tofu, cut into 4 slices
- 1 tbsp. olive oil
- ¼ cup oregano and parsley chimichurri

Directions:

1. In a small bowl, combine the oregano, cumin, coriander, and salt.
2. Sprinkle the spice rub on both sides of the tofu slices.
3. In a large nonstick skillet, heat the olive oil over medium-high heat until it shimmers.
4. Add the tofu and cook until browned, about 5 minutes per side.
5. Serve topped with the chimichurri.

Nutrition:

- Calories: 183
- Protein: 7 g
- Fats: 18 g
- Saturated Fat: 3 g
- Carbs: 2 g
- Fiber: 1 g
- Sodium: 479 mg

40. Grilled Eggplant Burgers

Preparation Time: 10 minutes
Cooking Time: 13 minutes
Servings: 2
Ingredients:

- 1 tbsp. olive oil
- 1 tsp. ground cumin
- 1 tsp. dried oregano
- ½ tsp. sea salt
- 2 (¼- to ½-inch-thick) eggplant slices
- 2 gluten-free hamburger buns
- ¼ cup lemon yogurt sauce

Directions:

1. Heat an indoor or outdoor grill to high.
2. In a small bowl, stir together the olive oil, cumin, oregano, and salt.
3. Brush the oil mixture on both sides of the eggplant slices. Brush any remaining mixture on the inside of the gluten-free buns.
4. Grill the eggplant slices for 5 to 6 minutes per side, or until browned.
5. Grill the buns until toasted, about 1 minute.
6. Assemble the burgers and serve topped with the yogurt sauce.

Nutrition:

- Calories: 237
- Protein: 3 g
- Fats: 13 g
- Saturated Fat: 2 g
- Carbs: 32 g
- Fiber: 7 g
- Sodium: 699 mg

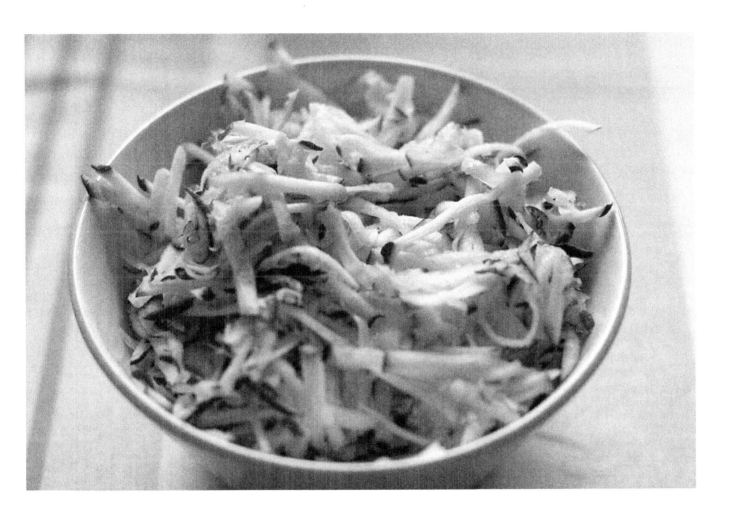

CAPITOLO 14:

Second Courses to Counter Acidity

1. Zucchini with Marinara and Cheese

Preparation Time: 10 minutes
Cooking Time: 25 minutes
Servings: 6
Ingredients:

- 1 cup panko
- ⅓ cup parmesan cheese, freshly grated
- Kosher salt and freshly ground black pepper, to taste
- 2 zucchinis, thinly sliced to ¼-inch-thick rounds
- ⅓ cup all-purpose flour
- 2 large eggs, beaten
- ½ cup marinara sauce
- ½ cup mozzarella pearls, drained
- 2 tbsp. fresh parsley leaves, chopped

Directions:

1. Preheat the broiler to 400°F. Daintily oil a sheet or coat it with nonstick cooking spray.
2. In an enormous bowl, consolidate the panko and parmesan, and season with salt and pepper, to taste. Set it aside.
3. Working in clumps, dig the zucchini in the flour, dunk it into the eggs, and dig it into the panko blend, squeezing to cover.
4. Spot the zucchini in a solitary layer onto the readied heating sheet. Place it on the stove and heat until delicate and brilliant dark-colored, about 18 to 20 minutes.
5. Top with marinara and mozzarella.
6. At that point cook for 2 to 3 minutes, or until the cheddar has dissolved.
7. Serve it quickly, embellished with parsley if desired.

Nutrition:

- Calories: 217
- Carbs: 21 g
- Fats: 12 g

2. Grilled Fig and Peach-Arugula Salad

Preparation Time: 10 minutes
Cooking Time: 20 minutes
Servings: 2
Ingredients:
For the Dressing:

- 3 tbsp. good-quality olive oil
- 1 tsp. good balsamic vinegar ½ lemon from juice
- Salt, to taste - 6–7 tsp freshly ground pepper

For the Salad:

- 4 figs, halved - 1 tsp. dark brown sugar
- Salt, to taste - Olive oil, to taste
- A few handfuls (2 oz.) arugula, cleaned and dried
- 1 yellow peach, sliced - 3–4 pistachios, chopped
- 2 prosciutto slices
- Ricotta salata, for serving

Directions:

1. In a little bowl, including the olive oil, balsamic vinegar, lemon juice, squeeze of salt, and naturally ground pepper; blend until well combined. Do a trial and include more salt, if you like. Put in a safe spot.
2. Sprinkle the figs with the brown sugar and a touch of salt. Start a barbecue or a broil skillet. When hot, brush with the olive oil. Place the figs on the broil skillet and cook for 1 minute, or until the barbecue imprints show up. Remove it from the heat and put it in a safe spot.
3. Place the arugula into a huge blending bowl. Sprinkle the leaves with salt. Add half of the dressing, and delicately prepare the serving of mixed greens. Move the lettuce to your serving plate. Add the peaches to the blending bowl and hurl with a touch of dressing. Move the peaches and figs to the serving plate, masterminding anyway you like. Top with a sprinkling of pistachios, a couple of torn bits of prosciutto, and small pieces of ricotta salata.

Nutrition:

- Calories: 3 Carbs: 26 g
- Fats: 24 g Protein: 10 g

3.   Lean Spring Stew

Preparation Time: 15 minutes
Cooking Time: 1 hour and 15 minutes
Servings: 4
Ingredients:

- 1 lb. tomatoes, diced and fire-roasted
- 4 boneless, skinless chicken thighs
- 1 tbsp. dried basil
- 8 oz. chicken stock
- Salt and pepper, to taste
- 4 oz. tomato paste
- 3 celery stalks, chopped
- 3 carrots, chopped
- 2 chili peppers, finely chopped
- 2 tbsp. olive oil
- 1 onion, finely chopped
- 2 garlic cloves, crushed
- ½ container mushrooms
- Sour cream, for serving

Directions:

1. Heat the olive oil over medium-high temperature. Add the celery, onions, and carrots. Then stir-fry for 5 minutes.
2. Transfer to a deep pot and add the tomato paste, basil, garlic, mushrooms, and seasoning. Keep stirring the vegetables until they are completely covered by tomato sauce. At the same time, cut the chicken into small cubes to make it easier to eat.
3. Put the chicken in a deep pot, pour the chicken stock over it, and throw in the tomatoes.
4. Stir the chicken in to ensure the ingredients and vegetables are properly mixed with it. Turn the heat to low and cook for about 1 hour. The vegetables and chicken should be cooked through before you turn the heat off. Top with sour cream and serve!

Nutrition:

- Calories: 277
- Carbs: 19 g
- Fiber: 3 g
- Fats: 11.9 g

4.   Yummy Chicken Bites

Preparation Time: 10 minutes
Cooking Time: 10 minutes
Servings: 2
Ingredients:

- 1 lb. chicken breasts, skinless, boneless, and cut into cubes
- 2 tbsp. fresh lemon juice
- 1 tbsp. fresh oregano, chopped
- 2 tbsp. olive oil
- ⅛ tsp. cayenne pepper
- Pepper, to taste
- Salt, to taste

Directions:

1. Place the chicken in a bowl.
2. Add the remaining ingredients over the chicken, and mix well.
3. Place the chicken in the refrigerator for 1 hour.
4. Heat the grill over medium heat.
5. Spray the grill with cooking spray.
6. Thread marinated chicken onto skewers.
7. Arrange the skewers on the grill and grill until chicken is cooked.
8. Serve and enjoy.

Nutrition:

- Calories: 560
- Fats: 31 g
- Carbs: 1.8 g
- Sugar: 0.4 g
- Protein: 66 g
- Cholesterol: 200 mg

5.   Shrimp Scampi

Preparation Time: 5 minutes
Cooking Time: 8 minutes
Servings: 4
Ingredients:

- 1 lb. shrimp
- ¼ tsp. red pepper flakes
- 1 tbsp. fresh lemon juice
- ¼ cup butter
- ½ cup chicken broth
- 2 garlic cloves, minced
- 1 shallot, sliced
- 3 tbsp. olive oil
- 3 tbsp. parsley, chopped
- Pepper, to taste
- Salt, to taste

Directions:

1. Heat the oil in a pan over medium heat.
2. Add the garlic and shallots and cook for 3 minutes.
3. Add the broth, lemon juice, and butter. Then cook for 5 minutes.
4. Add the red pepper flakes, parsley, pepper, and salt. Stir.
5. Add the shrimp and cook for 3 minutes.
6. Serve and enjoy.

Nutrition:

- Calories: 336
- Fats: 24 g
- Carbs: 3 g
- Sugar: 0.2 g
- Protein: 26 g
- Cholesterol 269 mg

6.   Zucchini Frittata

Preparation Time: 10 minutes
Cooking Time: 10 minutes
Servings: 4
Ingredients:

- 2 tsp. butter, divided
- 1 cup zucchini, shredded
- Salt and freshly ground black pepper, to taste
- 4 eggs, lightly beaten
- 2 tbsp. skim milk
- ¼ tsp. garlic salt
- ¼ tsp. onion powder
- 2 tbsp. mild Cheddar cheese, shredded

Directions:

1. In a medium nonstick skillet over medium heat, melt 1 tsp. butter and sauté the zucchini until softened and lightly browned, about 4 to 5 minutes, stirring frequently.
2. Drain the zucchini if necessary and season to taste with salt and pepper. Beat the eggs with milk, garlic, salt, onion powder, and zucchini until combined. Melt the remaining 1 teaspoon of butter in skillet, add egg mixture, and cook until partially set. Lift the edges of the cooked egg with a spatula, let the uncooked egg run underneath, and continue until the top of the frittata is set, about 4 minutes.
3. Carefully flip the frittata and let cook until lightly browned, about 4 minutes. Remove the skillet from the heat, sprinkle the cheese over the frittata, and let stand until cheese is melted.
4. Cut the frittata in half and serve immediately. Enjoy!

Nutrition:

- Calories: 20
- Fats: 15 g
- Saturated Fat: 7 g
- Protein: 14 g
- Carbs: 4 g
- Fiber: 1 g
- Sugar: 3 g

7.   Salmon Patties

Preparation Time: 10 minutes
Cooking Time: 10 minutes
Servings: 3
Ingredients:

- 1 (14 ½-oz.) can salmon
- 4 tbsp. butter
- 1 avocado, diced
- 2 eggs, lightly beaten
- ½ cup almond flour
- ½ onion, minced
- Pepper, to taste
- Salt, to taste

Directions:

1. Add all the ingredients except the butter in a large mixing bowl, and mix until well combined.
2. Make 6 patties from the mixture. Set aside.
3. Melt the butter in a pan over medium heat.
4. Place the patties on a pan and cook for 5 minutes on each side.
5. Serve and enjoy.

Nutrition:

- Calories: 9
- Fats: 49 g
- Carbs: 11 g
- Sugar: 2 g
- Protein: 36 g
- Cholesterol: 225 mg

8.   Apple Cinnamon Oatmeal

Preparation Time: 10 minutes
Cooking Time: 5 minutes
Servings: 1
Ingredients:

- ½ cup skim milk
- ⅓ cup water
- 1 apple (peeled, cored, and diced)
- A dash of salt
- ½ cup old fashioned oats
- ¼ tsp. cinnamon
- ¼ tsp. vanilla

Directions:

1. Mix the milk, water, apple, and salt in a small saucepan. Heat the mixture to a simmer, stirring occasionally (do not boil).
2. Add the oats and cinnamon to saucepan and simmer, uncovered, for about 5 minutes, stirring occasionally.
3. Stir the vanilla into the oatmeal and serve immediately. Enjoy!

Nutrition:

- Calories: 18
- Fats: 2 g
- Saturated Fat: 0 g
- Protein: 7 g
- Carbs: 36 g
- Fiber: 4 g
- Sugar: 19 g

9.   Stuff Cheese Pork Chops

Preparation Time: 10 minutes
Cooking Time: 35 minutes
Servings: 4
Ingredients:

- 4 pork chops, boneless and thickly cut
- 2 tbsp. olives, chopped
- 2 tbsp. sun-dried tomatoes, chopped
- ½ cup feta cheese, crumbled
- 2 garlic cloves, minced
- 2 tbsp. fresh parsley, chopped

Directions:

1. Preheat the oven to 375°F.
2. In a bowl, mix the feta cheese, garlic, parsley, olives, and sun-dried tomatoes.
3. Stuff the feta cheese mixture in the pork chops. Season with the pepper and salt.
4. Bake for 35 minutes.
5. Serve and enjoy.

Nutrition:

- Calories: 31
- Fats: 25 g
- Carbs: 2 g
- Sugar: 1 g
- Protein: 21 g
- Cholesterol: 75 mg

10.   Italian Pork Chops

Preparation Time: 10 minutes
Cooking Time: 30 minutes
Servings: 4
Ingredients:

- 4 pork loin chops, boneless
- 2 garlic cloves, minced
- 1 tsp. Italian seasoning
- 1 tbsp. fresh rosemary, chopped
- ¼ tsp. black pepper
- ½ tsp. kosher salt

Directions:

1. Season the pork chops with pepper and salt.
2. In a small bowl, mix the garlic, Italian seasoning, and rosemary.
3. Rub the pork chops with the garlic and rosemary mixture.
4. Place the pork chops on a baking tray and roast them in the oven at 350°F for 10 minutes.
5. Turn temperature to 325°F and roast the chops for 25 minutes more
6. Serve and enjoy.

Nutrition:

- Calories: 261
- Fats: 19 g
- Carbs: 2 g
- Sugar: 0 g
- Protein: 18 g
- Cholesterol: 68 mg
- Fiber: 0.4 g
- Carbs: 1 g

11.   Sunshine Wrap

Preparation Time: 10 minutes
Cooking Time: 30 minutes
Servings: 2
Ingredients:

- 8 oz. grilled chicken breast
- ½ cup celery, diced
- ⅔ cup mandarin oranges
- ¼ cup onion, minced
- 2 tbsp. mayonnaise
- 1 tsp. soy sauce
- ¼ tsp. garlic powder
- ¼ tsp. black pepper
- 1 whole wheat tortilla
- 4 lettuce leaves

Directions:

1. Combine all the ingredients, except the tortilla and lettuce, in a large bowl and toss to coat evenly.
2. Lay the tortillas on a flat surface, and cut them into quarters.
3. Top each quarter with a lettuce leaf, and spoon the chicken mixture into the middle of each leaf.
4. Roll each tortilla into a cone and seal by slightly wetting the edge with water. Enjoy!

Nutrition:

- Calories: 280.8
- Fats: 21.1 g
- Carbs: 3 g
- Protein: 19 g

12.   Taco Omelet

Preparation Time: 10 minutes
Cooking Time: 10 minutes
Servings: 1
Ingredients:

- 2 eggs, lightly beaten
- 2 tbsp. skim milk
- ¼ tsp. chili powder
- ¼ tsp. garlic powder
- ¼ tsp. onion powder
- Salt and freshly ground black pepper, to taste
- 1 tsp. vegetable oil
- 1 tbsp. guacamole
- 1 tbsp. sour cream
- 1 tbsp. salsa
- 2 tbsp. Cojack cheese, shredded

Directions:

1. In a medium bowl, whisk the eggs, milk, chili powder, garlic powder, and onion powder. Then season to taste with salt and pepper.
2. Heat the oil in a medium nonstick skillet over medium heat. Pour the egg mixture into the skillet and swirl to coat evenly. Cover the skillet and let the eggs cook until set on top, about 4 minutes.
3. With a large spatula, carefully flip the omelet. Season the omelet to taste with salt and pepper and let cook until lightly browned on the bottom, about 6 minutes more.
4. Slide the omelet onto a plate. Spread the guacamole, sour cream, and salsa all over one side of the omelet and sprinkle with cheese. Fold the omelet in half over the filling and serve immediately. Enjoy.

Nutrition:

- Calories: 290
- Fats: 22 g
- Saturated Fat: 10 g
- Protein: 17 g
- Carbs: 6 g
- Fiber: 1 g
- Sugar: 3 g

13. Sheet Pan Spicy Tofu and Green Beans

Preparation Time: 10 minutes
Cooking Time: 30 minutes
Servings: 4
Ingredients:

- 1 tsp. garlic, minced
- ¼ cup scallions, sliced
- 2 tsp. sesame seeds, plus more for garnish
- 3 tbsp. soy sauce
- 1 tbsp. sesame oil
- 1 tsp. red pepper flakes
- ½ tsp. maple syrup
- 2 tbsp. rice wine vinegar
- 16 oz. firm tofu, drained and pressed
- 1 oz. green beans, trimmed
- 2 tsp. olive oil, for oiling the pan
- Salt and pepper, to taste

Directions:

1. Preheat the broiler to 400°F.
2. Flush and channel the tofu, and press utilizing a tofu press, and place the dish on top. Let it boil through 10 to 15 minutes, this will enable the marinades to be integrated.
3. Whisk together the ingredients for the zesty sauce.
4. Cut the tofu into triangles and place them in a single layer on a previously oiled sheet. Cover it with the hot sauce and cook for 12 minutes.
5. Flip the tofu and sprinkle with more sauce. Add the green beans to the opposite side of the container in a single layer. Cover with the residual sauce and sprinkle with salt and pepper.
6. Return it to the stove and heat it until it is caramelized and somewhat fresh, about 12–15 minutes.
7. Sprinkle with the residual sesame seeds, whenever wanted, and serve.

Nutrition:

- Calories: 21
- Carbs: 20 g
- Fats: 11 g
- Protein: 12 g

14. Skillet Chicken Thighs with Potato, Apple, and Spinach

Preparation Time: 10 minutes
Cooking Time: 20 minutes
Servings: 1
Ingredients:

- 1 small chicken thigh
- Salt, to taste
- Pepper, to taste
- 1 tsp. canola oil
- 1 medium russet potato, cut into ½ inch cubes
- 1 small fuji apple, cored and cut into 6 wedges
- 1 tsp. fresh sage, chopped
- 1 cup packed baby spinach

Directions:

1. Heat the broiler to 400°F.
2. Season the chicken generously with salt and pepper.
3. Heat the oil in a large, broiler-secure skillet over medium heat. Place the chicken skin-side down and prepare the dinner till pores and skin crisps marginally and a few fats are extracted. Add the potato, apple, and sage. Toss to cowl and arrange potato and apple around the skillet, making sure it is skin-side down.
4. Place the skillet in the broiler and leave it there for 15 minutes. Flip the chicken and broil for 10 extra minutes, or until the potatoes and apples are delicate and the chicken is cooked through with no red within the middle.
5. Return the skillet to the stovetop over medium-low heat. Remove the chicken with spinach, and toss with potatoes and apples to shrink.
6. Top vegetable mixture with chicken to serve.

Nutrition:

- Calories: 514
- Fats: 22 g
- Carbs: 59 g
- Sugar: 23 g
- Protein: 21 g

15. Cherry Tomatoes Tilapia Salad

Preparation Time: 10 minutes
Cooking Time: 25 minutes
Servings: 3
Ingredients:

- 1 cup mixed greens
- 1 cup cherry tomatoes
- ⅓ cup red onion, diced
- 1 medium avocado
- 3 tortilla crusted tilapia fillet

Directions:

1. Spray the tilapia fillet with a little bit of cooking spray. Put the fillets in the air fryer basket. Cook for 24 minutes at about 390°F.
2. Transfer the fillet to a bowl. Toss with the tomatoes, greens, and red onion. Add the lime dressing and mix again.
3. Serve and enjoy!

Nutrition:

- Calories: 271
- Fats: 8 g
- Carbs: 10.1 g
- Protein: 18.5 g

16. Apple Cider Glazed Chicken Breast with Carrots

Preparation Time: 10 minutes
Cooking Time: 6 hours 45 minutes
Servings: 2
Ingredients:

- 2 boneless, skin-on chicken breasts
- 2 cups apple cider
- 4 whole peppercorns
- 2 small bunches fresh sage
- ½ tsp. salt
- 2 tbsp. olive oil
- Salt and pepper, to taste
- 4 carrots, peeled and sliced
- 1 tbsp. butter

Directions:

1. To start with, in all probability, the boneless, skin-on chicken bosom still has the tenderloin connected. Remove it. (It's the additional piece that resembles a chicken strip). This helps the chicken cook quicker. I solidify the tenderloins for soup or make chicken strips with them.
2. In a large dish or bowl, add the chicken, apple juice, peppercorns, sage (torn and hacked first), and ½ teaspoon of salt. Let it marinate shrouded in the cooler for at least 4 hours.
3. Following 4 hours, remove the chicken and pat the chicken dry. Heat the oil in a large skillet. At the point when the oil is hot, sprinkle the chicken with additional salt and pepper, and place it skin-side down in the container. Cook on both sides until it becomes darker.
4. In the meantime, strip and bone the carrots. Spot them in a microwave-safe bowl, spread them with the saran wrap, and microwave them for 1 minute.
5. Take the flavors out from the apple juice, and after that, pour it over the chicken once the two sides becomes dark colored. Adjust the heat so that the apple juice goes to a stew and cooks until the chicken reaches 16°F on a thermometer. Remove the chicken and put it aside when done.
6. When the chicken is done, turn the heat to high and lessen the apple juice to a thick coat. Add the carrots and sauté them for 3 to 4 minutes, or until fresh delicate. Add the spread before removing them from the dish. Mix to cover the carrots in the coating and margarine. Utilize any additional coating from the dish to brush on the chicken, and serve the chicken with the carrots.

Nutrition:

- Calories: 328 Fats: 20 g Carbs: 39 g
- Sugar: 2 Protein: 2 g

17. Onion Paprika Pork Tenderloin

Preparation Time: 10 minutes
Cooking Time: 3 hours 10 minutes
Servings: 6
Ingredients:

- 2 lbs. pork tenderloin

For the Rub:

- 1 ½ tbsp. smoked paprika
- 1 tbsp. garlic powder
- 1 ½ tbsp. onion powder
- ½ tbsp. salt

Directions:

1. Preheat the oven to 425°F.
2. In a small bowl, mix all the rub ingredients and rub over the pork tenderloin.
3. Spray a pan with cooking spray and heat it over medium-high heat.
4. Sear the pork on all sides until lightly golden brown.
5. Place the pan into the oven and roast the pork for about 3 hours 10 minutes.
6. Slice and serve.

Nutrition:

- Calories: 225
- Fats: 5 g
- Carbs: 2 g
- Sugar: 1 g
- Protein: 41 g
- Cholesterol: 45 mg

18. Rosemary Garlic Pork Chops

Preparation Time: 10 minutes
Cooking Time: 35 minutes
Servings: 4
Ingredients:

- 4 pork chops, boneless
- ¼ tsp. onion powder
- 2 garlic cloves, minced
- 1 tsp. dried rosemary, crushed
- ¼ tsp. pepper
- ¼ tsp. sea salt

Directions:

1. Preheat the oven to 425°F.
2. Season the pork chops with onion powder, pepper, and salt.
3. Mix the rosemary and garlic, and then rub the mixture over the pork chops.
4. Place the pork chops on a baking tray and roast for 10 minutes.
5. Set the temperature to 350°F and roast for 25 minutes more.
6. Serve and enjoy.

Nutrition:

- Calories: 260
- Fats: 20 g
- Carbs: 1 g
- Sugar: 0 g
- Protein: 19 g
- Cholesterol: mg

19.   Skinny Chicken Pesto Bake

Preparation Time: 10 minutes
Cooking Time: 20 minutes
Servings: 4
Ingredients:

- 160 oz. skinless chicken
- 1 tsp. basil
- 1 tomato, sliced
- 6 tbsp. mozzarella cheese, shredded
- 2 tsp. parmesan cheese, grated

Directions:

1. Cut the chicken into thin strips.
2. Set the oven to 400°F. Prepare a baking sheet by lining it with parchment paper.
3. Lay the chicken strips on a prepared baking sheet. Top with the pesto and brush evenly over the chicken pieces.
4. Set to bake until chicken is fully cooked (about 15 minutes).
5. Garnish with parmesan cheese, mozzarella, and tomatoes.
6. Set to continue baking until the cheese melts (about 5 minutes).

Nutrition:

- Calories: 205
- Fats: 8.5 g
- Carbs: 2.5 g
- Protein: 30 g

20.   Cold Tomato Couscous

Preparation Time: 10 minutes
Cooking Time: 10 minutes
Servings: 4
Ingredients:

- 5 oz. couscous
- 3 tbsp. tomato sauce
- 3 tbsp. lemon juice
- 1 small-sized onion, chopped
- 1 cup vegetable stock
- ½ small-sized cucumber, sliced
- ½ small-sized carrot, sliced
- ¼ tsp. salt
- 3 tbsp. olive oil
- ½ cup fresh parsley, chopped

Directions:

1. First, pour the couscous into a large bowl. Boil the vegetable broth and slightly add in the couscous while stirring constantly. Leave it for about minutes, or until the couscous absorbs the liquid. Cover with a lid and set aside. Stir from time to time to speed up the soaking process and break the lumps with a spoon.
2. Meanwhile, preheat the olive oil in a frying pan, and add the tomato sauce. Add the chopped onion and stir until translucent. Set aside and let it cool for a few minutes.
3. Add the oily tomato sauce to the couscous and stir well. Now add the lemon juice, chopped parsley, and salt to the mixture and give it a final stir.
4. Serve with the sliced cucumber, carrot, and parsley.

Nutrition:

- Carbs: 32.8 g
- Fiber: 3.2 g
- Fats: 11 g
- Calories: 249

21.   Fresh Shrimp Rolls

Preparation Time: 10 minutes
Cooking Time: 20 minutes
Servings: 12
Ingredients:

- 12 sheets rice paper
- 12 bib lettuces
- 12 basil leaves
- ¾ cup cilantro
- 1 cup carrots, shredded
- ½ cucumber, sliced
- 20 oz. cooked shrimp
- Water, as needed

Directions:

1. Add all the vegetables and shrimp to separate the bowls.
2. Set a damp paper towel tower flat on the work surface.
3. Quickly wet a sheet of rice paper under warm water and lay it on a paper towel.
4. Top with 1 of each vegetable and 4 pieces of shrimp, then roll it in the rice paper into a burrito.
5. Repeat until all the vegetables and the shrimp have been used up. Serve and enjoy.

Nutrition:

- Calories: 67
- Fats: 2.9 g
- Carbs: 7.4 g
- Protein: 2.6 g

22.   Chicken Breast Tortilla

Preparation Time: 10 minutes
Cooking Time: 30 minutes
Servings: 2
Ingredients:

- 8 oz. grilled chicken breast
- ½ cup celery, diced
- ⅔ cup mandarin oranges
- ¼ cup minced onion
- 2 tbsp. mayonnaise
- 1 tsp. soy sauce
- ¼ tsp. garlic powder
- ¼ tsp. black pepper
- 1 whole wheat tortilla
- 4 lettuce leaves

Directions:

1. Combine all the ingredients, except the tortilla and lettuce, in a large bowl and toss to coat evenly.
2. Lay the tortillas on a flat surface and cut them into quarters.
3. Top each quarter with a lettuce leaf and spoon some chicken mixture into the middle of each.
4. Roll each tortilla into a cone and seal by slightly wetting the edge with water. Enjoy!

Nutrition:

- Calories: 280.8
- Fats: 21.1 g
- Carbs: 3 g
- Protein: 19 g

23. Sweet Roasted Beet and Arugula Tortilla Pizza V

Preparation Time: 10 minutes
Cooking Time: 10 minutes
Servings: 6
Ingredients:

- 2 beets, chopped
- 6 tortillas, corn
- 1 cup arugula
- ½ c. goat cheese
- 1 cup blackberries
- 2 tbsp. honey
- 2 tbsp. balsamic vinegar

Directions:

1. Preheat the oven to 350°F. Lay the tortillas on a flat surface.
2. Top with the beets, berries, and goat cheese. Combine the balsamic vinegar and honey in a small bowl, and whisk to combine.
3. Drizzle the mixture over the pizza to bake for about 10 minutes, or until cheese has melted slightly and the tortilla is crisp.
4. Garnish with the arugula and serve.

Nutrition:

- Calories: 286
- Fats: 40 g
- Carbs: 42 g
- Protein: 15 g

24. Southwestern Black Bean Cakes with Guacamole

Preparation Time: 10 minutes
Cooking Time: 25 minutes
Servings: 4
Ingredients:

- 1 cup whole wheat bread crumbs
- 3 tbsp. cilantro, chopped
- 2 garlic cloves
- 15 oz. black beans
- 7 oz. chipotle peppers in adobo sauce
- 1 tsp. ground cumin
- 1 large egg
- ½ avocado, diced
- 1 tbsp. lime juice
- 1 tomato plum

Directions:

1. Drain the beans and add all the ingredients, except avocado, lime juice, and eggs, to a food processor and run it until the mixture begins to pull away from the sides.
2. Transfer to a large bowl and add the egg, then mix well.
3. Form into 4 even patties and cook on a preheated, greased grill over medium heat for about 10 minutes, flipping halfway through.
4. Add the avocado and lime juice in a small bowl, then stir and mash together using a fork.
5. Season to taste then serve with bean cakes.

Nutrition:

- Calories: 178
- Fats: 7 g
- Carbs: 25 g
- Protein: 11 g

25. Veggie Quesadillas with Cilantro Yogurt Dip

Preparation Time: 10 minutes
Cooking Time: 25 minutes
Servings: 3
Ingredients:

- 1 cup black beans
- 2 tbsp. chopped cilantro
- ½ bell pepper, chopped
- ½ cup corn kernels
- 1 cup cheese, shredded
- 6 corn tortillas
- 1 carrot, shredded

Directions:

1. Set skillet to preheat on low heat. Lay 3 tortillas on a flat surface.
2. Top evenly with the peppers, carrots, cilantro, beans, corn, and cheese over the tortillas, covering each with another tortilla.
3. Add the quesadilla to the preheated skillet. Cook until the cheese melts and the tortillas are golden brown, about 2 minutes.
4. Flip the quesadilla and cook for about 1 minute, or until golden.
5. Mix well. Slice each quesadilla into 4 even wedges and serve with dip. Enjoy!

Nutrition:

- Calories: 344 Fats: 8 g
- Carbs: 46 g Protein: 27 g

26. Mayoless Tuna Salad

Preparation Time: 5 minutes
Cooking Time: 10 minutes
Servings: 2
Ingredients:

- 5 oz. tuna
- 1 tbsp. olive oil
- 1 tbsp. red wine vinegar
- ¼ cup green onion, chopped
- 2 cup arugula
- 1 cup cooked pasta
- 1 tbsp. parmesan cheese
- Black pepper, to taste

Directions:

1. Combine all the ingredients into a medium bowl. Split the mixture between 2 plates. Serve and enjoy.

Nutrition:

- Calories: 213.2 - Fats: 6.2 g
- Carbs: 20.3 g
- Protein: 22.7 g

27. Southwest Style Zucchini Rice Bowl

Preparation Time: 10 minutes
Cooking Time: 12 minutes
Servings: 2
Ingredients:

- 1 tbsp. vegetable oil
- 1 cup vegetables, chopped
- 1 cup chicken breast, chopped
- 1 cup zucchini rice, cooked
- 4 tbsp. salsa
- 2 tbsp. cheddar cheese, shredded
- 2 tbsp. sour cream

Directions:

1. Set a skillet with oil to heat up over medium heat.
2. Add the chopped vegetables and allow to cook, stirring until the vegetables become fork tender.
3. Add the chicken and zucchini rice. Cook while stirring until fully heated through.
4. Split between the 2 serving bowls and garnish with the remaining ingredients. Serve and enjoy!

Nutrition:

- Calories: 168
- Fats: 8.2 g
- Carbs: 18 g
- Protein: 5.5 g

28. Pesto and Mozzarella Stuffed Portobello Mushroom Caps

Preparation Time: 10 minutes
Cooking Time: 15 minutes
Servings: 2
Ingredients:

- 2 Portobello mushrooms
- 1 Roma tomato, diced
- 2 tbsp. pesto
- ¼ cup mozzarella cheese, shredded

Directions:

1. Spoon the pesto evenly into the mushroom caps, then top with the remaining ingredients.
2. Bake at 400°F for about 15 minutes. Enjoy!

Nutrition:

- Calories: 112
- Fats: 5.4 g
- Carbs: 7.5 g
- Protein: 10.5 g

29. Tandoori Chicken

Preparation Time: 10 minutes
Cooking Time: 35 minutes
Servings: 6
Ingredients:

- 1 cup plain yogurt
- ½ cup lemon juice
- 5 garlic cloves, crushed
- 2 tbsp. paprika
- 1 tsp. yellow curry powder
- 1 tsp. ground ginger
- 6 skinless chicken breasts
- 6 skewers

Directions:

1. Set oven to 400°F. In a blender, combine the red pepper flakes, ginger, curry, paprika, garlic, lemon juice, and yogurt, then process into a smooth paste.
2. Add the chicken strips evenly onto skewers. Add the chicken to a shallow casserole dish, then cover with ½ of the yogurt mixture.
3. Seal it tightly and let it rest in the refrigerator for about 15 minutes.
4. Lightly grease a baking tray, then transfer the chicken skewers onto it, and top with the remaining yogurt mixture.
5. Set to bake until the chicken is fully cooked. Serve and enjoy.

Nutrition:

- Calories: 177
- Fats: 7.2 g
- Carbs: 6 g
- Protein: 20.6 g

30. Turkey Fajitas Bowls

Preparation Time: 10 minutes
Cooking Time: 5 minutes
Servings: 4
Ingredients:

- ½ lb. turkey breast
- 2 tbsp. olive oil
- 1 tbsp. lemon juice
- 1 garlic, crushed
- ¾ tsp. chili pepper, chopped
- ½ tsp. dried oregano
- 1 bell pepper, sliced
- 1 medium tomato
- ½ cup cheddar cheese, shredded
- 4 tostada bowls
- 4 tbsp. salsa

Directions:

1. Add the oregano, chili pepper, garlic, lemon juice, and 1 tablespoon of olive oil to a medium bowl. Whisk to combine.
2. Add the turkey then toss to coat. Allow marinating for about 30 minutes.
3. Set a skillet over medium heat with the remaining oil. Add bell pepper and allow it to cook for 2 minutes while stirring.
4. Add the turkey and cook for 3 more minutes. Add the tomato, stir, and remove from heat.
5. Spoon the mixture evenly into the tostada bowls.
6. Garnish with the cheese and salsa then serve.

Nutrition:

- Calories: 240
- Fats: 15 g
- Carbs: 5 g
- Protein: 23 g

31.   Baked Chicken Pesto

Preparation Time: 10 minutes
Cooking Time: 30 minutes
Servings: 4
Ingredients:

- 160 oz. skinless chicken
- 1 tsp. basil
- 1 tomato, sliced
- 6 tbsp. mozzarella cheese, shredded
- 2 tsp. parmesan cheese, grated
- 2 tbsp Pesto

Directions:

1. Set oven to 400°F. Prepare a baking sheet by lining it with parchment paper.
2. Lay the chicken strips on the prepared baking sheet. Top with pesto and brush evenly over chicken pieces.
3. Set to bake until the chicken is fully cooked, about 15 minutes.
4. Garnish with parmesan cheese, mozzarella, and tomatoes.
5. Set to continue baking until the cheese melts, about 5 minutes.

Nutrition:

- Calories: 205
- Fats: 8.5 g
- Carbs: 2.5 g
- Protein: 30 g

32.   Spaghetti Squash Lasagna V

Preparation Time: 10 minutes
Cooking Time: 25 minutes
Servings: 6
Ingredients:

- 2 cups marinara sauce
- 3 cups spaghetti squash, roasted
- 1 cup ricotta
- 8 tsp. parmesan cheese, grated
- 6 oz. mozzarella cheese, shredded
- ¼ tsp. red pepper flakes

Directions:

1. Set the oven to preheat to 375°F and spoon half of the marinara sauce into a baking dish.
2. Top with the squash, then layer the remaining ingredients.
3. Cover and set to bake until the cheeses are melted and the edges brown, about 20 minutes.
4. Remove the cover and bake for another 5 minutes. Enjoy!

Nutrition:

- Calories: 255
- Fats: 15.9 g
- Carbs: 5.5 g
- Protein: 21.4 g

33. Crab Mushrooms

Preparation Time: 10 minutes
Cooking Time: 5 minutes
Servings: 5
Ingredients:

- 5 oz. crab meat
- 5 oz. white mushrooms
- ½ tsp. salt
- ¼ cup fish stock
- 1 tsp. butter
- ¼ tsp. ground coriander
- 1 tsp. dried cilantro
- 1 tsp. butter

Directions:

1. Chop the crab meat and sprinkle with the salt and dried cilantro.
2. Mix the crab meat carefully. Preheat the air fryer to 400°F.
3. Chop the white mushrooms and combine them with the crab meat.
4. Add the fish stock, ground coriander, and butter.
5. Transfer the side dish mixture into the air fryer basket tray.
6. Stir gently with the help of a plastic spatula.
7. Cook the side dish for 5 minutes.
8. Rest for 5 minutes. Serve and enjoy!

Nutrition:

- Calories: 56
- Fats: 1.7 g
- Carbs: 2.6 g
- Protein: 7 g

34. Loaded Sweet Potatoes

Preparation Time: 15 minutes
Cooking Time: 35 minutes
Servings: 4
Ingredients:

- 4 medium sweet potatoes, baked
- ½ cup Greek yogurt
- 1 tsp. taco seasoning
- 1 tsp. olive oil
- 1 red pepper, diced
- ½ red onion, diced
- 1 ⅓ cups canned black beans
- ½ cup Mexican cheese blend
- ¼ cup cilantro, chopped
- ½ cup salsa

Directions:

1. Mix the taco seasoning and yogurt well, then set aside.
2. Set a skillet over medium heat with oil to get hot.
3. Add in the remaining ingredients, except the potatoes, cheese, and salsa. Then cook for about 8 minutes, or until fully heated through.
4. Slightly pierce the potatoes down the center, and top evenly with all remaining ingredients. Serve.

Nutrition:

- Calories: 311
- Fats: 8.3 g
- Carbs: 57 g
- Protein: 3.2 g

35. Coconut Flour Spinach Casserole

Preparation Time: 10 minutes
Cooking Time: 30 minutes
Servings: 6
Ingredients:

- 4 eggs
- ¾ cup unsweetened almond milk
- 3 oz. spinach, chopped
- 3 oz. artichoke hearts, chopped
- 1 cup parmesan, grated
- 3 garlic cloves, minced
- 1 tsp. salt
- ½ tsp. pepper
- ¾ cup coconut flour
- 1 tbsp. baking powder
- Basil, chopped, for serving

Directions:

1. Preheat the air fryer to 375°F. Grease the air fryer's pan with cooking spray.
2. Whisk the eggs with almond milk, spinach, artichoke hearts, and ½ cup of parmesan cheese. Add the salt, garlic, and pepper.
3. Add the coconut flour and baking powder; whisk until well combined.
4. Spread the mixture into the air fryer pan, and sprinkle the remaining cheese over it.
5. Place the baking pan in the air fryer and cook for about 30 minutes.
6. Remove the baking pan from the air fryer, and sprinkle with chopped basil. Slice, then serve and enjoy!

Nutrition:

- Calories: 175.2
- Fats: 10.3 g
- Carbs: 2.4 g
- Protein: 17.7 g

36. Tilapia with Cherry Tomatoes

Preparation Time: 10 minutes
Cooking Time: 18 minutes
Servings: 3
Ingredients:

- 1 cup mixed greens
- 1 cup cherry tomatoes
- ⅓ cup red onion, diced
- 1 medium avocado
- 3 tortilla crusted tilapia fillet

Directions:

1. Spray the tilapia fillet with a little bit of cooking spray. Put the fillets in the air fryer basket. Cook at about 390°F for 18 minutes.
2. Transfer the fillet to a bowl. Toss with the tomatoes, greens, and red onion. Add the lime dressing, and mix again.
3. Serve and enjoy!

Nutrition:

- Calories: 271
- Fats: 8 g
- Carbs: 10.1 g
- Protein: 18.5 g

37.   Strawberry Frozen Yogurt Squares

Preparation Time: 10 minutes
Cooking Time: 8 hours
Servings: 8
Ingredients:

- 1 cup barley and wheat cereal
- 3 cups fat-free strawberry yogurt
- 10 oz. frozen strawberries
- 1 cup fat-free milk
- 1 cup whipped topping

Directions:

1. Set a parchment paper on the baking tray.
2. Spread the cereal evenly over the bottom of the tray.
3. Add the milk, strawberries, and yogurt to a blender, and process into a smooth mixture.
4. Use the yogurt mixture to top the cereal, wrap with foil, and place to freeze until firm (about 8 hours).
5. Let it thaw lightly, slice it into squares, and serve.

Nutrition:

- Calories: 188
- Fats: 0 g
- Carbs: 43.4 g
- Protein: 4.6 g

38.   Smoked Tofu Quesadillas

Preparation Time: 10 minutes
Cooking Time: 5 minutes
Servings: 4
Ingredients:

- 1 lb. extra-firm sliced tofu
- 12 tortillas
- 2 tbsp. coconut oil
- 6 cheddar cheese, slices
- 2 tbsp. sundried tomatoes
- 5 tbsp. sour cream

Directions:

1. Lay one tortilla flat and fill it with the tofu, tomato, and cheese. Then top it with the oil. Repeat for as many as you need.
2. Bake for 5 minutes and remove from heat.
3. Top with the sour cream.

Nutrition:

- Calories: 136
- Fats: 6 g
- Carbs: 13 g
- Protein: 10 g

39.   Zucchini Pizza Boats

Preparation Time: 10 minutes
Cooking Time: 45 minutes
Servings: 2
Ingredients:

- 2 medium zucchini
- ½ cup tomato sauce
- ½ cup mozzarella cheese, shredded
- 2 tbsp. Parmesan cheese

Directions:

1. Set oven to 350°F.
2. Slice the zucchini in half lengthwise, and spoon out the core and seeds to form boats.
3. Place the zucchini halves skin-side down in a small baking dish.
4. Add the remaining ingredients inside the hollow center, then set to bake until golden brown and fork-tender, about 30 minutes.
5. Serve and enjoy.

Nutrition:

- Calories: 214 - Fats: 7.9 g
- Carbs: 23.6 g - Protein: 15.2 g

40.   Pear-Cranberry Pie with Oatmeal Streusel

Preparation Time: 10 minutes
Cooking Time: 1 hour and 30 minutes
Servings: 6
Ingredients:
For the Streusel:

- ¾ cup oats
- ⅓ cup stevia
- ½ tsp. cinnamon
- ¼ tsp. nutmeg
- 1 tbsp. butter, cubed

For the Filling:

- 3 cups pears, cubed
- 2 cups cranberries - ½ cup stevia
- 2 ½ tbsp. cornstarch

Directions:

1. Set the oven to 350°F.
2. Combine all the streusel ingredients in a food processor, and process into a coarse crumb.
3. Next, combine all the filling ingredients in a large bowl, and toss to combine.
4. Transfer the filling into the pie crust, then top with the streusel mixture.
5. Set to bake until golden brown, about 1 hour. Let cool and serve.

Nutrition:

- Calories: 280 Fats: 9 g
- Carbs: 47 g - Protein: 1 g

41.   Mixed Sweet Potatoes

Preparation Time: 15 minutes
Cooking Time: 8 minutes
Servings: 2
Ingredients:

- 4 medium sweet potatoes, baked
- 1 tsp. taco seasoning
- 1 tsp. olive oil
- 1 red pepper, diced
- ½ red onion, diced
- 1 ⅓ cup canned black beans
- ½ cup Mexican cheese blend
- ½ cup Greek yogurt
- ¼ cup cilantro, chopped
- ½ cup salsa

Directions:

1. Mix the taco seasoning and yogurt well, then set aside.
2. Set a skillet over medium heat with oil to get hot.
3. Add in the remaining ingredients, except the potatoes, cheese, and salsa. Then cook for about 8 minutes, or until fully heated through.
4. Slightly pierce the potatoes down the center, and top evenly with all remaining ingredients. Serve.

Nutrition:

- Calories: 311
- Fats: 6
- Carbs: 15
- Protein: 4
- Sodium: 155

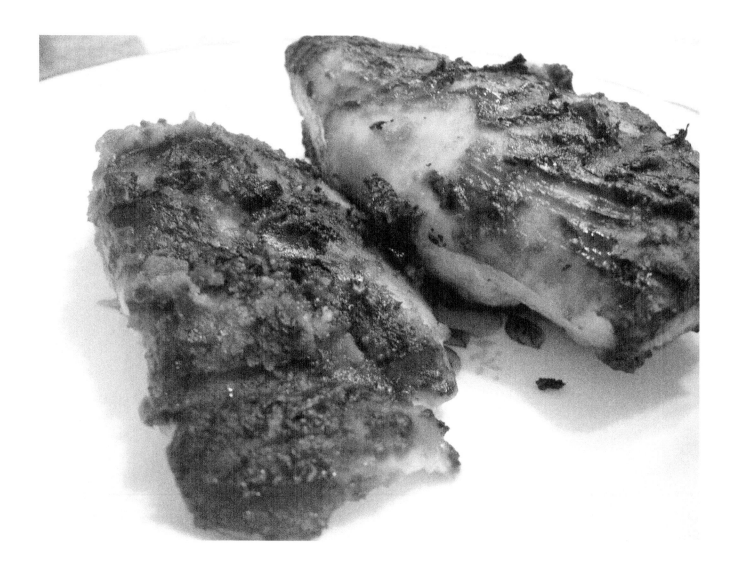

CAPITOLO 15:

Side Dishes to Protect the Gastric Mucous Membranes

1. Skillet Peanut Butter Cinnamon Spice Cookie

Preparation Time: 20 minutes
Cooking Time: 10–12 minutes
Servings: 16
Ingredients:

- 1 large egg
- 1 cup natural peanut butter
- ½ cup brown sugar
- ¼ cup almond meal
- 1 tsp. vanilla extract
- 1 tsp. baking soda
- 1 tsp. cinnamon
- ¼ tsp. ground ginger
- ¼ tsp. salt
- Nonstick spray
- 2 tbsp. peanuts, optional, for garnish

Directions:

1. Preheat the oven to 350°F.
2. In a large bowl, beat the egg until slightly frothy. Whisk in the peanut butter, brown sugar, almond meal, vanilla extract, baking soda, cinnamon, ginger, and salt until well combined.
3. Spray an oven-proof skillet lightly with nonstick spray. Pour the batter into the skillet and spread evenly with a spatula. If desired, sprinkle the top with a few peanuts and press down slightly.
4. Place the cookie on a rack set in the center of the oven and bake for 10–12 minutes, or until puffed and golden around the edges. Let cool 10 minutes before cutting and serving.

Nutrition:

- Calories: 129
- Fats: 10 g
- Carbs: 8 g
- Protein: 5 g

2. Turkey Burger Salad with Avocado to Cure Acid Reflux

Preparation Time: 20 minutes
Cooking Time: 4–5 minutes
Servings: 4
Ingredients:

- 1 oz. ground turkey, formed into 4 patties (preferably 93% lean/7% fat, as 99% lean can be too dry)
- ½ tsp. sea salt
- 2 romaine lettuce heads, washed and cut, or torn into 2- to 3-inch pieces
- 1 medium-size can small black olives, pitted
- 2 tbsp. extra-virgin olive oil
- 1 tsp. balsamic vinegar
- 1 avocado, peeled and sliced

Directions:

1. Season the turkey patties with the salt, and then cook on the grill or the stovetop in a covered frying pan over medium to medium-high heat for 4 to 5 minutes per side.
2. After cooking, put the burgers aside until cool enough to break into bite-size pieces.
3. Place the lettuce, olives, oil, and vinegar in a large salad bowl and toss.
4. Finally, add the burger pieces and avocado slices on top.

Nutrition:

- Calories: 364
- Calories from Fats: 129
- Fats: 13 g
- Saturated Fat: 12 g
- Trans Fats: 0 g
- Cholesterol: 67 mg
- Sodium: 378 mg

3. Rice Noodle Medley

Preparation Time: 5 minutes
Cooking Time: 30 minutes
Servings: 6
Ingredients:

- 1 cup rice uncooked
- 1 tbsp. butter
- 1 ½ cups medium noodles
- 3 cup chicken or vegetable broth
- Salt and pepper, to taste

Directions:

1. In a large nonstick pot coated with nonstick cooking spray, brown the rice in butter, stirring.
2. Add the noodles, broth, salt, and pepper. Bring the mixture to boil, reduce heat, and cook covered for 20–30 minutes, or until the rice and noodles are done.

Nutrition:

- Calories: 174
- Protein: 5 g
- Carbs: 32 g
- Fats: 2 g
- Calories from Fats: 10%
- Saturated Fat: 0 g
- Dietary Fiber: 1 g
- Cholesterol: 11 mg
- Sodium: 341 mg

4. Chicken and Red Potatoes Recipe

Preparation Time: 15 minutes
Cooking Time: 50 minutes
Servings: 4
Ingredients:

- 10 ½ oz. red potatoes cut into one-inch cubes
- 2 large carrots, peeled and sliced into 1-inch pieces
- 1 tbsp. grass-fed butter melted
- ¼ tsp. kosher salt
- ¼ tsp. turmeric
- 2 cups grilled chicken meat, shredded or chopped
- ½ tsp. dried rosemary
- ⅓ cup green olives, pitted (optional)
- 2 tbsp. organic apple cider vinegar
- 2 tbsp. fresh parsley
- 2 limes, cut into thin slices

Directions:

1. Preheat the oven to 425°F.
2. Toss the potatoes and carrots together with the melted butter, salt, and turmeric. Spread evenly onto a rimmed baking sheet. Squeeze the juice out of limes and add them to the baking sheet. Bake until the vegetables are tender, about 35 minutes, stirring halfway through the cooking.
3. Transfer the roasted red potatoes and carrots to a casserole dish, and then stir in chicken, rosemary, olives, and apple cider vinegar.
4. Cook for 15 more minutes, or until heated through.
5. Garnish with the parsley and serve hot.

Nutrition:

- Calories: 412
- Calories from Fats: 198
- Fats: 22 g
- Saturated Fat: 7 g
- Sodium: 940 mg
- Potassium: 787 mg
- Carbs: 19 g
- Dietary Fiber: 4 g
- Sugar: 3 g
- Protein: 34 g

5. Absolute Coconut Balls

Preparation Time: 20 minutes
Cooking Time: 10 minutes
Servings: 8
Ingredients:

- ½ cup coconut water (liquid from coconut)
- 3 cups coconut milk
- 3 tbsp. coconut flakes
- 1 cup coconut flour
- 1 tsp. pure vanilla extract (no alcohol)
- ½ tsp. salt
- Stevia sweetener, granulated to taste
- ½ cup. coconut, shredded

Directions:

1. Boil the coconut water, coconut milk, coconut flour, coconut flakes, salt, and stevia in a saucepan over medium-low heat.
2. Cook until the mixture achieves a creamy consistency.
3. Allow it to cool completely, add the vanilla extract, and stir well.
4. Shape the balls and roll them in the shredded coconut.
5. Place the coconut balls on a platter lined with parchment paper.
6. Refrigerate for 3 to 4 hours.
7. Serve.

Nutrition:

- Calories: 131,82
- Fats: 11 g
- Saturated Fat: 10 g
- Cholesterol: 0 mg
- Carbs: 7 g
- Protein: 28 g

6. Fried Seasoned Cabbage

Preparation Time: 15 minutes
Cooking Time: 0 minutes
Servings: 8
Ingredients:

- 2 tbsp. olive oil
- ½ cabbage head, chopped
- 1 tbsp. cilantro, chopped
- Kosher salt, to taste
- 1 tbsp. cider vinegar
- 1 tbsp. cumin seeds
- 1 tsp. tarragon

Directions:

1. Heat the oil into a large nonstick skillet over medium heat.
2. Add the cabbage, salt, and cilantro. Stir with the spatula for 30 seconds.
3. Keep stirring until the edges are lightly charred.
4. Drizzle with the cider vinegar and stir until combined well.
5. Taste and adjust the salt to taste.
6. Sprinkle with the cumin and tarragon. Serve.

Nutrition:

- Calories: 277
- Fats: 14 g
- Saturated Fat: 2 g
- Cholesterol: 0 mg
- Sodium: 83 mg
- Dietary Fiber: 8 g
- Sugar: 12 g
- Protein: 8 g

7.   Potato Medley Soup

Preparation Time: 5 minutes
Cooking Time: 15 minutes
Servings: 4
Ingredients:

- 3 cups stock
- 1 tbsp. oil
- ⅔ lb. potato
- Fresh herbs, for serving
- ½ lb. raw vegetables, chopped

Directions:

1. Sauté the vegetables with the potatoes in a greased cooking pot until soft.
2. Stir in the stock and bring it to a simmer.
3. Cook for 15 minutes, and then blend until smooth.
4. Serve warm with fresh herbs on top.

Nutrition:

- Calories: 304
- Fats: 30.6 g
- Carbs: 21.4 g
- Protein: 4.6 g

8.   Vegetable Soup

Preparation Time: 10 minutes
Cooking Time: 35 minutes
Servings: 4
Ingredients:

- ¼ tsp. golden caster sugar
- 3 tbsp. olive oil
- 2 rosemary sprig
- 1 carrot, chopped
- 1 celery stick, chopped
- 3 cups vegetable stock
- 2 bay leaves
- ½ lb. cauliflower florets
- ¼ lb. white cabbage, shredded
- ½ lb. gluten-free sourdough bread, sliced
- 1 tbsp. caraway seeds
- 1 potato, chopped
- 1 tsp. Worcestershire sauce

Directions:

1. Set the oven to 320°F to preheat.
2. Spread the bread baking tray along with caraway seeds, sea salt, and 1 tablespoon of oil.
3. Bake for 10 minutes, or until golden.
4. In a large pot, add the carrot, potato, and the remaining olive oil.
5. Cook for 5 minutes, or until soft.
6. Stir in the celery, seasoning, sugar, stock, bay leaves, thyme, and rosemary.
7. Boil the mixture, then reduce the heat to a simmer.
8. Cook for 10 minutes, and then add the cabbage and cauliflower.
9. Cook for another 15 minutes, or until al dente.
10. Stir in the Worcestershire sauce.
11. Discard the bay leaves, thyme, and rosemary. Serve warm.

Nutrition:

- Calories: 418
- Fats: 3.8 g
- Carbs: 13.3 g
- Protein: 5.4 g

9. Spaghetti with Watercress and Pea Pesto

Preparation Time: 5 minutes
Cooking Time: 6 minutes
Servings: 4
Ingredients:

- ¼ cup watercress
- ¼ cup vegetarian fat-free hard cheese
- 3 ¼ cups wholemeal spaghetti
- 2 egg whites
- 2 tbsp. olive oil
- 2 cups frozen peas

Directions:

1. Heat the water to a simmer in a cooking pan, and then add the peas.
2. Cook for 3 minutes, drain, and then set it aside.
3. Blend the peas with watercress and cheese until it forms into a thick paste.
4. Add the olive oil and blend again until smooth.
5. Meanwhile, boil the spaghetti as per the given instructions, then drain and keep it aside.
6. Add the water to a suitable cooking pot and bring it to simmer.
7. Create a whirlpool in the water, and add the egg whites into it. Cook for 3 minutes.
8. Mix the pesto with the spaghetti, and serve with the poached egg whites and the watercress on top.

Nutrition:

- Calories: 341
- Fats: 4 g
- Carbs: 16.4 g
- Protein: 0.3 g

10. Cran-Apple Carrot Muffins

Preparation Time: 15 minutes
Cooking Time: 40 minutes
Servings: 12
Ingredients:

- 1 ¼ cups whole wheat flour
- ½ cup brown sugar
- ½ tsp. baking powder
- ½ tsp. baking soda
- 1 tsp. cinnamon
- ½ tsp. salt
- 1 cup rolled oats
- 1 tbsp. ground flaxseed
- 2 ½ tbsp. water
- 3 tbsp. olive oil
- ⅓ cup non-fat plain Greek yogurt
- ½ cup applesauce
- 4 medium carrots, grated (about 1 ¾ to 2 cups)
- ½ cup fresh cranberries, roughly chopped

Directions:

1. Preheat oven to 400°F. Spray a 12-cup muffin tin with cooking spray, and set it aside.
2. Whisk together the flour, sugar, baking powder, baking soda, cinnamon, and salt. Stir in the oats.
3. In a small bowl, mix the ground flaxseed with the water. Let it sit for at least 5 minutes for it to start to gel (this acts as an egg in the recipe).
4. Add the olive oil, yogurt, and applesauce to the "flax egg," and whisk together. Dump the mixture into the dry ingredients along with the carrots and cranberries.
5. Using a rubber spatula, stir until the mixture is just combined. Do not overmix; otherwise, the muffins will come out tough.
6. Spoon the batter evenly among the muffin tin and bake for 24 to 28 minutes, or until the tops are puffed and golden and a toothpick inserted in the center comes out clean. Let cool on a wire rack.

Nutrition:

- Calories: 309
- Fats: 9 g
- Saturated Fat: 1 g
- Cholesterol: 0 mg
- Sodium: 381 mg
- Carbs: 53 g
- Dietary Fiber: 7 g
- Sugar: 21 g
- Protein: 7 g

11.   Simple Vegetable Broth

Preparation Time: 5 minutes
Cooking Time: 2 hours
Servings: 8
Ingredients:

- 2 carrots, peeled and chopped
- 1 leek, green part only, chopped and washed
- 1 celery stalk, chopped
- 1 fennel bulb, chopped
- 9 cups water

Directions:

1. In a large pot, combine all the ingredients.
2. Bring to a simmer over medium-high heat, then lower the heat to low and simmer for 2 hours.
3. Strain the vegetables from the broth, and store the broth until you're ready to use it.

Nutrition:

- Calories: 1
- Protein: 0 g
- Fats: 0 g
- Carbs: 3 g

12.   Miso Soup with Tofu and Greens

Preparation Time: 5 minutes
Cooking Time: 8 minutes
Servings: 4
Ingredients:

- 1 leek, green part only, chopped and washed
- 3 oz. extra-firm tofu, cubed
- 7 cups simple vegetable broth, divided
- 3 cups baby spinach
- 2 tbsp. miso paste

Directions:

1. In a large nonstick pot, add the leek and tofu, then cook while stirring occasionally until the leek is soft, about 5 minutes.
2. Add 6 cups of broth. Bring to a simmer and lower the heat to medium.
3. Add the spinach. Cook for 3 minutes.
4. In a small bowl, whisk together the remaining 1 cup of broth and the miso paste. Stir into the hot soup. Stir-cook for 30 seconds more. Serve.

Nutrition:

- Calories: 117
- Protein: 8 g
- Fats: 6 g
- Carbs: 12 g

13.   Italian Vegetable Soup

Preparation Time: 5 minutes
Cooking Time: 12 minutes
Servings: 4
Ingredients:

- 1 leek, green part only, chopped and washed
- 1 carrot, peeled and chopped
- 1 cup green beans, trimmed and chopped
- 1 cup canned kidney beans 1 zucchini, chopped
- 1 tbsp. dried Italian seasoning - ½ tsp. sea salt
- 7 cups simple vegetable broth
- 2 tbsp. fresh basil, chopped

Directions:

1. In a large nonstick pot, add the leek, carrot, and zucchini. Then cook while stirring occasionally until the leek is soft, about 5 minutes.
2. Add the green beans, kidney beans, Italian seasoning, salt, and vegetable broth. Bring to a simmer, then lower the heat to medium. Simmer while stirring occasionally until the green beans are tender, about 5 to 7 minutes.
3. Stir in the basil before serving.

Nutrition:

- Calories: 120 - Protein: 5 g
- Fats: 4 g - Carbs: 18 g

14.   Creamy Pumpkin Soup

Preparation Time: 5 minutes
Cooking Time: 12 minutes
Servings: 4
Ingredients:

- 1 leek, green part only, washed and finely chopped - 1 cup canned pure pumpkin
- 3 cups simple vegetable broth - 1 tsp. dried sage
- ½ tsp. sea salt - ½ cup light coconut milk, nonfat
- 1 tsp. cornstarch

Directions:

1. In a large saucepan, add the leek and stir-cook until soft, about 5 minutes.
2. Add the pumpkin, vegetable broth, sage, and salt. Bring to a simmer and cook for 5 minutes.
3. In a small bowl, whisk together the coconut milk and cornstarch. Remove the pan from the heat, and carefully pour the soup into a blender or food processor along with the coconut milk and cornstarch. Allow the steam to escape through the hole in the blender lid or the food processor feed tube as you blend to avoid a buildup of pressure. Blend until smooth.
4. Return the soup to the pot and warm it over medium heat for 2 minutes, or until thick. Serve.

Nutrition:

Calories: 92 Protein: 2 g Fats: 5 g Carbs: 10 g

15.   Cream of Broccoli Soup

Preparation Time: 5 minutes
Cooking Time: 10 minutes
Servings: 4
Ingredients:

- 1 green leek, finely chopped and washed
- 3 cups broccoli florets
- 6 cups simple vegetable broth
- ½ tsp. sea salt
- 1 cup lactose-free nonfat milk
- 1 tbsp. cornstarch
- ½ cup baby kale
- ¼ cup microgreens

Directions:

1. In a large pot, add the leek and broccoli and stir-cook until the leek is soft, about 5 minutes.
2. Add the vegetable broth and salt. Bring to a simmer. Lower the heat to medium and simmer while stirring occasionally until the broccoli is soft, about 5 minutes.
3. In a small bowl, whisk together the milk and cornstarch. Stir into the soup. Cook for a few minutes more, stirring until the soup thickens slightly.
4. Garnish with the kale and microgreens (if using), and serve.

Nutrition:

- Calories: 127
- Protein: 6 g
- Fats: 4 g
- Carbs: 19 g

16.   Roasted Veggie and Goat Cheese Frittata

Preparation Time: 15 minutes
Cooking Time: 30 minutes
Servings: 6
Ingredients:

- ½ medium zucchini, diced in medium pieces
- ½ cup small broccoli florets
- 1 medium carrot, diced into small pieces
- ½ small sweet potato, diced into small pieces
- ½ cup baby bella mushrooms, sliced
- 1 tsp. basil
- ½ tsp. thyme
- 1 tsp. oregano
- ¼ tsp. salt
- 1 tbsp. olive oil
- 4 large eggs
- ⅛ tsp. turmeric
- ¼ cup goat cheese, crumbled

Directions:

1. Preheat oven to 350°F.
2. Add all of the chopped vegetables to a greased 9-inch cake pan and toss with basil, thyme, oregano, salt, and olive oil. Roast for about 15 to 20 minutes, or until the sweet potato and carrots are softened.
3. Meanwhile, in a small bowl, whisk together the eggs, turmeric, and crumbled goat cheese.
4. Remove the vegetables from the oven and use a spoon to distribute them throughout the pan evenly.
5. Pour the egg mixture over the vegetables and cook for another 5 to 10 minutes, or until the eggs are set.
6. Remove from oven and let cool. Slice and serve!

Nutrition:

- Calories: 110
- Fats: 5 g
- Carbs: 7 g
- Protein: 7 g

17. Mini Pizzas with Spinach and White Sauce

Preparation Time: 10 minutes
Cooking Time: 12 minutes
Servings: 4
Ingredients:

- 4 oz. premade raw pizza dough
- All-purpose flour, for dusting
- ½ cup low-fat white sauce
- ¼ cup fat-free Parmesan cheese, grated
- 1 tsp. dried Italian seasoning
- 1 cup fresh baby spinach, divided
- 8 mushrooms, sliced, divided
- 4 oz. fat-free mozzarella cheese, grated, divided
- 4 tbsp. fresh basil, chopped

Directions:

1. Preheat the oven to 400°F.
2. Divide the dough into 4 pieces. On a floured surface, roll each piece into a round that is about ⅜-inch thick. Place the rounds on a nonstick baking sheet.
3. In a small bowl, whisk the white sauce and Parmesan cheese together. Spread each pizza with 2 tablespoons of sauce. Sprinkle with the Italian seasoning.
4. Top each with ¼ cup of spinach, one-fourth of the mushrooms, and 1 ounce of mozzarella cheese.
5. Bake for about 12 minutes, or until the dough is golden and the cheese has melted.
6. Serve garnished with the basil.

Nutrition:

- Calories: 234
- Fats: 7 g
- Saturated Fat: 3 g
- Cholesterol: 16 mg
- Carbs: 16 g
- Fiber: 2 g
- Protein: 12 g
- Sodium: 801 mg

18. Mushroom Stroganoff

Preparation Time: 10 minutes
Cooking Time: 12 minutes
Servings: 4
Ingredients:

- 2 tbsp. extra-virgin olive oil
- 12 oz. shiitake mushrooms, sliced
- 1 tsp. dried thyme
- ½ tsp. sea salt
- 3 cups mushroom broth
- 3 tbsp. arrowroot powder
- 1 tbsp. Dijon mustard
- ½ cup fat-free sour cream
- ¼ cup fresh parsley, chopped
- 6 oz. egg noodles, cooked according to package directions and drained

Directions:

1. In a 12-inch nonstick sauté pan or skillet over medium-high heat, heat the oil until it shimmers.
2. Add the mushrooms, thyme, and salt. Cook for 4 minutes without stirring. Continue to cook for 4 minutes more, stirring occasionally.
3. In a small bowl, whisk together the broth, arrowroot powder, and mustard until smooth. Stir this into the mushrooms. Cook for about 2 minutes, stirring constantly until thick and warmed through.
4. Stir in the sour cream and parsley. Cook for 1 to 2 minutes, stirring constantly.
5. Serve over the hot egg noodles.

Nutrition:

- Calories: 250
- Fats: 8 g
- Saturated Fat: 1 g
- Cholesterol: 15 mg
- Carbs: 30 g
- Fiber: 2 g
- Protein: 8 g
- Sodium: 488 mg

19. Fettuccine Alfredo

Preparation Time: 15 minutes
Cooking Time: 4 minutes
Servings: 4
Ingredients:

- 3 cups (1 recipe) low-fat white sauce
- 1 cup cooked peas
- ¼ cup fat-free Parmesan cheese, grated
- 6 oz. fettuccine noodles, cooked according to package directions and drained
- 2 tbsp. fresh basil, chopped

Directions:

1. In a medium saucepan over medium heat, simmer the white sauce, peas, and Parmesan cheese for 4 minutes, stirring constantly.
2. Toss the sauce with the hot noodles and fresh basil.

Nutrition:

- Calories: 201
- Fats: 2 g
- Saturated Fat: 1 g
- Cholesterol: 37 mg
- Carbs: 33 g
- Fiber: 2 g
- Protein: 12 g
- Sodium: 160 mg

20. Veggie Tacos

Preparation Time: 10 minutes
Cooking Time: 15 minutes
Servings: 4
Ingredients:

- 4 corn tortillas
- 2 tbsp. extra-virgin olive oil
- 2 carrots, peeled and grated
- 1 zucchini, chopped
- 4 oz. mushrooms, finely chopped
- 1 tsp. ground cumin
- ½ tsp. ground coriander
- 1 tsp. sea salt, divided
- ½ cup black beans, drained and heated
- ¼ cup fresh cilantro, chopped
- 2 oz. fat-free cheddar cheese, grated
- ½ cup fat-free sour cream
- ½ tsp. grated lime zest

Directions:

1. Preheat the oven to 350°F.
2. Wrap the tortillas in aluminum foil and place them in the oven to warm for about 15 minutes, or until heated through.
3. Meanwhile, in a large nonstick sauté pan or skillet over medium-high heat, heat the oil until it shimmers.
4. Add the carrots, zucchini, mushrooms, cumin, coriander, and ½ teaspoon of salt. Cook for about 5 minutes, stirring occasionally until the vegetables begin to brown.
5. In a medium bowl, mash the black beans, cilantro, and the remaining ½ teaspoon of salt. Spread the bean mixture on the hot tortillas.
6. Top each tortilla with one-fourth of the cooked vegetables and sprinkle with cheddar cheese.
7. In a small bowl, mix the sour cream and lime zest. Dollop on the tacos.

Nutrition:

- Calories: 236
- Fats: 8 g
- Saturated Fat: 1 g
- Cholesterol: 6 mg
- Carbs: 31 g
- Fiber: 5 g
- Protein: 10 g
- Sodium: 622 mg

21. Artichoke Purée

Preparation Time: 10 minutes
Cooking Time: 5 minutes
Servings: 6
Ingredients:

- 1 (14-oz.) can artichoke bottoms, drained
- ½ cup lactose-free, nonfat milk, or non-dairy milk (such as rice milk)
- 1 tbsp. unsalted, grass-fed butter
- ½ tsp. sea salt

Directions:

1. In a small saucepan, combine all the ingredients. Cook over medium-high heat, stirring occasionally until warm, about 5 minutes.
2. Transfer to a blender or food processor and blend until smooth.

Nutrition:

- Calories: 134
- Protein: 4 g
- Fats: 10 g
- Saturated Fat: 2 g
- Carbs: 12 g
- Fiber: 4 g
- Sodium: 694 mg

22. Green Beans Amandine

Preparation Time: 10 minutes
Cooking Time: 4 minutes
Servings: 6
Ingredients:

- ¼ cup slivered almonds
- 24 green beans, trimmed and halved
- 1 tbsp. olive oil
- ½ tsp. lemon zest, grated
- ½ tsp. sea salt

Directions:

1. Preheat the oven to 350°F.
2. Spread the almonds in a single layer on a rimmed baking sheet and bake until toasted, about 5 minutes.
3. Fill a large pot halfway with water and bring to a boil over high heat. Add the beans and cook covered until tender, about 4 minutes. Drain.
4. Toss the beans with the toasted almonds, olive oil, lemon zest, and sea salt.

Nutrition:

- Calories: 185 Protein: 5 g
- Fats: 16 g Saturated Fat: 2 g
- Carbs: 8 g
- Fiber: 4 g
- Sodium: 591 mg

23. Roasted Asparagus with Goat Cheese

Preparation Time: 5 minutes
Cooking Time: 15 minutes
Servings: 6
Ingredients:

- 10 asparagus spears
- 1 tbsp. olive oil
- ½ tsp. sea salt
- 2 tbsp. goat cheese, crumbled
- ½ tsp. lemon zest, grated

Directions:

1. Preheat the oven to 425°F.
2. On a rimmed baking sheet, toss the asparagus with the olive oil and sea salt. Bake for 15 minutes, or until tender.
3. Sprinkle with the goat cheese and lemon zest before serving.

Flavor Boost: toast ¼ cup of the walnut pieces in a 350°F oven for 5 minutes, and sprinkle over the asparagus for a toasty flavor and a nice crunch.

Nutrition:

- Calories: 94 Protein: 3 g
- Fats: 8 g Saturated Fat: 2 g
- Carbs: 3 g Fiber: 2 g
- Sodium: 609 mg

24. Creamed Spinach

Preparation Time: 5 minutes
Cooking Time: 10 minutes
Servings: 6
Ingredients:

- 1 tbsp. olive oil
- 1 bunch spinach, stemmed and chopped
- ½ tsp. sea salt
- A pinch ground nutmeg
- ½ cup lactose-free, nonfat milk
- 1 tsp. cornstarch

Directions:

1. In a large pot, heat the olive oil over medium-high heat until it shimmers. Add the spinach, salt, and nutmeg. Cook until the spinach is wilted, about 3 minutes.
2. In a small bowl, whisk together the milk and cornstarch. Add to the spinach. Stir-cook until the milk thickens, about 1 minute.

Substitution: This also works well with greens such as kale, collards, or Swiss chard. Cooking these greens may take longer, about 5 to 7 minutes.

Nutrition:

- Calories: 135 Protein: 7 g Fats: 8 g Saturated
- Fat: 1 g Carbs: 13 g Fiber: 4 g Sodium: 748 mg

25. Mashed Potatoes

Preparation Time: 10 minutes
Cooking Time: 15 minutes
Servings: 6
Ingredients:

- 2 russet potatoes, peeled and cut into ½-inch cubes
- ½ cup lactose-free nonfat milk
- 2 tbsp. unsalted grass-fed butter, at room temperature
- ½ tsp. sea salt

Directions:

1. Put the potatoes in a large pot and cover them with plenty of water. Cover and cook over high heat until the potatoes are soft, about 15 minutes. Drain the potatoes and return them to the pot.
2. Add the milk, butter, and salt. Mash with a potato masher until smooth. Taste for seasoning and add more salt if necessary.

Substitution: You can also use this recipe to make mashed potatoes. Replace the russet potatoes with 4 unpeeled red potatoes, cut them into ½-inch cubes. The skins will give extra texture to the potatoes.

Nutrition:

- Calories: 136
- Protein: 3 g
- Fats: 6 g
- Saturated Fat: 4 g
- Carbs: 21 g
- Fiber: 1 g
- Sodium: 313 mg

26. Quinoa Pilaf

Preparation Time: 10 minutes
Cooking Time: 20 minutes
Servings: 6
Ingredients:

- 1 tbsp. olive oil
- 1 carrot, peeled and chopped
- ½ cup quinoa, rinsed
- 1 cup simple vegetable broth (here)
- ¼ cup pine nuts
- 2 tbsp. raisins
- 2 tbsp. fresh parsley, chopped
- ½ tsp. sea salt

Directions:

1. In a medium pot, heat the oil over medium-high heat until it shimmers. Add the carrot and cook, stirring occasionally, until it starts to brown, about 5 minutes.
2. Add the quinoa and vegetable broth. Reduce to a simmer, cover, and cook until the quinoa is soft, about 15 minutes.
3. Add the pine nuts, raisins, parsley, and salt just before serving.

Nutrition:

- Calories: 171
- Protein: 4 g
- Fats: 8 g
- Saturated Fat: 1 g
- Carbs: 23 g
- Fiber: 3 g
- Sodium: 369 mg

27. Roasted Honey-Ginger Carrots

Preparation Time: 5 minutes
Cooking Time: 20 minutes
Servings: 4
Ingredients:

- 4 large carrots, peeled and cut lengthwise into quarters
- 2 tbsp. honey
- 1 tbsp. olive oil
- 1 tsp. fresh ginger, grated
- ½ tsp. salt

Directions:

1. Preheat the oven to 425°F.
2. Put the carrots in a single layer on a rimmed baking sheet.
3. In a small bowl, whisk together the honey, olive oil, ginger, and salt.
4. Drizzle over the carrots, turning to coat.
5. Bake until the carrots are tender, about 20 minutes.

Nutrition:

- Calories: 186 Protein: 1 g
- Fats: 7 g Saturated Fat: 1 g
- Carbs: 32 g Fiber: 4 g Sodium: 682 mg

28. Chopped Kale Salad

Preparation Time: 15 minutes
Cooking Time: 0 minutes
Servings: 2
Ingredients:

- 2 cups kale, stemmed and chopped
- 3 radishes, chopped
- 1 carrot, peeled and chopped
- ¼ cup lactose-free, nonfat plain yogurt
- 1 tsp. Dijon mustard
- 1 tsp. fresh thyme, chopped
- 1 tsp. fresh dill, chopped
- ½ tsp. orange zest, grated
- ½ tsp. sea salt

Directions:

1. In a large bowl, toss together the kale, radishes, and carrot.
2. In a small bowl, whisk together the yogurt, mustard, thyme, dill, orange zest, and sea salt.
3. Toss the dressing with the salad to serve.

Nutrition:

- Calories: 73 Protein: 4 g
- Fats: <1 g Saturated Fat: <1 g Carbs: 13 g
- Fiber: 3 g Sodium: 687 mg

29. Quick Pasta Salad

Preparation Time: 15 minutes
Cooking Time: 0 minutes
Servings: 2
Ingredients:

- 2 cups gluten-free elbow macaroni, cooked
- 1 cup baby spinach
- ¼ cup canned chickpeas
- ¼ cup black olives, sliced
- ¼ cup fresh basil, chopped
- 1 cup Creamy Herbed Dressing

Directions:

1. In a large bowl, toss together the macaroni, spinach, chickpeas, olives, and basil.
2. Toss with the dressing.

Nutrition:

- Calories: 152 Protein: 7 g
- Fats: 2 g Saturated Fat: <1 g
- Carbs: 27 g Fiber: 4 g
- Sodium: 222 mg

30. Sprout Onion Fry

Preparation Time: 15 minutes
Cooking Time: 10 minutes
Servings: 8
Ingredients:

- 2 ½ lb. Brussels sprouts, trimmed
- 4 bacon slices, cut into 1-inch pieces
- 1 tbsp. extra-virgin coconut oil
- 1 tomato, chopped
- 1 onion, chopped
- 4 thyme or savory sprigs, divided
- 1 tsp. iodine-free Celtic sea salt
- Freshly ground pepper, to taste
- 2 tsp. lemon juice (optional)

Directions:

1. Add the sprouts to the boiling water in a stockpot.
2. Let them cook for about 3 to 5 minutes.
3. Drain and set them aside.
4. Sauté the onions in a greased skillet for 4 minutes. Stir in salt, pepper, and thyme
5. Add the drained sprouts to the skillet and stir cook for 3 minutes.
6. Remove and discard the herb sprigs.
7. Serve warm with the lemon juice and the chopped spring onion on top.

Nutrition:

- Calories: 383 Fats: 5.3 g
- Saturated Fat: 3.9 g Cholesterol: 135 mg
- Sodium: 487 mg Carbs: 76.8 g Fiber: 0.1 g
- Sugar: 0 g Protein: 27.7 g

31.   Veggies with Mushrooms

Preparation Time: 5 minutes
Cooking Time: 10 minutes
Servings: 4
Ingredients:

- 1 tsp. coconut oil
- 1 cup mushroom, sliced
- ½ cup onion, chopped
- 2 tbsp. garlic, smashed
- 2 tbsp. ginger, finely chopped
- 1 ½ tbsp. Sambal Oelek®
- 1 ½ cups cabbage, chopped
- 2 cups leeks, white part only, chopped
- ½ cup celery, chopped
- 2 tbsp. jalapeños, sliced
- ¼ cup green bell peppers, sliced
- 3 tbsp. vegetable stock

Directions:

1. Sauté the mushrooms and onion in a greased skillet for 3 minutes.
2. Stir in the ginger, garlic, and Sambal Oelek®. Then sauté for 30 seconds.
3. Add the cabbage, leeks, and peppers. Then cook for 2 minutes.
4. Adjust the seasoning with salt and pepper.
5. Add the vegetable stock and cook for 1 minute.
6. Serve warm.

Nutrition:

- Calories: 398
- Fats: 13.8 g
- Saturated Fat: 5.1 g
- Cholesterol: 200 mg
- Sodium: 272 mg
- Carbs: 13.6 g
- Fiber: 1 g
- Sugar: 1.3 g
- Protein: 51.8 g

32.   Green Bean Stir Fry

Preparation Time: 10 minutes
Cooking Time: 5 minutes
Servings: 2
Ingredients:

- 2 tbsp. unseasoned rice vinegar
- 1 lb. green beans, trimmed and cut into pieces
- 1 tbsp. grapeseed oil
- 1 tsp. red pepper flakes
- Celtic sea salt, iodine free
- 2 garlic cloves, crushed
- Freshly ground black pepper, to taste
- 2 tbsp. coconut oil
- 1 piece of ginger, minced

Directions:

1. Add the coconut oil and green bean to the skillet, and sauté for 2 to 3 minutes.
2. Stir in the ginger and garlic. Cook for 2 minutes.
3. Add all the remaining ingredients.
4. Serve warm.

Nutrition:

- Calories: 372
- Fats: 11.8 g
- Saturated Fat: 4.4 g
- Cholesterol: 62 mg
- Sodium: 1871 mg
- Carbs: 31.8 g
- Fiber: 0.6 g
- Sugar: 27.3 g
- Protein: 34 g

33. Rosemary Roasted Yams

Preparation Time: 10 minutes
Cooking Time: 50 minutes
Servings: 4
Ingredients:

- 2 cups yams, cubed
- 1 tbsp. coconut oil
- 6 fresh rosemary sprigs, leaves removed and finely chopped stems discarded
- Celtic sea salt, iodine-free, to taste
- Black pepper, to taste

Directions:

1. Preheat the oven to 375°F.
2. Mix the yams with the rosemary and oil in a bowl.
3. Spread the yams on a baking sheet.
4. Bake for 45 to 50 minutes.
5. Adjust the seasoning with salt and pepper.
6. Serve warm.

Nutrition:

- Calories: 341
- Fats: 34 g
- Saturated Fat: 8.5 g
- Cholesterol: 69 mg
- Sodium: 547 mg
- Carbs: 36.4 g
- Fiber: 1.2 g
- Sugar: 1 g
- Protein: 20.3 g

34. Peach Panzanella

Preparation Time: 10 minutes
Cooking Time: 4 minutes
Servings: 2
Ingredients:

- 3 shallots, finely sliced into rings
- 2 tbsp. cider vinegar
- 3 firm peaches, halved
- 3 ½ tbsp. coconut oil
- 1 pinch red chili flakes
- 1 pinch fennel seeds
- ½ lemon, juiced
- A handful Wild Rocket® small pack basil, leaves picked
- 1 cup cherry tomatoes, halved

Directions:

1. Toss the peaches with coconut oil, fennel seeds, chili flakes, and seasoning in a bowl.
2. Heat a pan over high heat and add the peaches to cook for 2 minutes per side.
3. Place the peaches on a plate. Set them aside.
4. Mix the shallots with the vinegar, coconut oil, and seasoning in a bowl.
5. Stir in capers, basil, and tomato, and lemon juice.
6. Toss in the peaches.
7. Serve.

Nutrition:

- Calories: 311
- Fats: 25.5 g
- Saturated Fat: 12.4 g
- Cholesterol: 69 mg
- Sodium: 58 mg
- Carbs: 1.4 g
- Fiber: 0.7 g
- Sugar: 0.3 g
- Protein: 18.4 g

35. Cabbage with Coconut and Sweet Potato

Preparation Time: 10 minutes
Cooking Time: 10 minutes
Servings: 2
Ingredients:

- 1 lb. sweet potatoes, unpeeled and halved
- 2 tbsp. coconut oil
- A pinch asafoetida
- 1 tsp. black mustard seeds
- 1 tsp. cumin seeds
- 2 dried red chilies
- 1 fresh red or green chili, seeds removed and thinly sliced
- 1 head cabbage, finely shredded
- ½ lemon, juiced
- 2 tbsp. fresh coconut, desiccated or shaved
- 2 cups Water, as needed
- 1 tbsp Salt, to taste
- 2 tbsp Coriander

Directions:

1. Add the water and salt to a large pot and boil it.
2. Stir in the potatoes and cook for 10 minutes.
3. Drain and transfer them to a bowl. Crush them with a fork gently (do not mash).
4. Heat the oil in a large skillet and add the spices, asafoetida, and chilies.
5. Sauté for 2 minutes and toss in the cabbage, fresh chili, and salt.
6. Stir-cook for about 3 to 4 minutes.
7. Stir in the drained potatoes and cook for 2 to 3 minutes.
8. Add the coconut, coriander, and lemon juice
9. Mix well and serve warm with the coconut yogurt.

Nutrition:

- Calories: 604
- Fats: 30.6 g
- Saturated Fat: 13.1 g
- Cholesterol: 131 mg
- Sodium: 1834 mg
- Carbs: 21.4 g
- Fiber: 0.2 g
- Sugar: 20.3 g
- Protein: 54.6 g

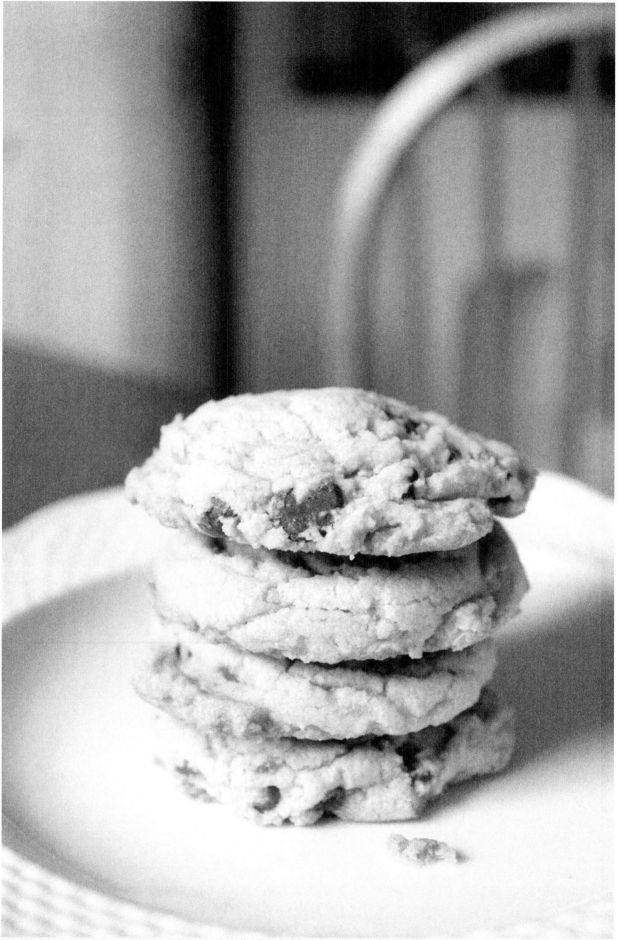

CAPITOLO 16:

Sweets Not to Burden the Stomach

1.   Vanilla Pudding

Preparation Time: 5 minutes
Cooking Time: 10 minutes
Servings: 6
Ingredients:

- 2 ¼ cups nonfat milk, divided
- 1 tsp. vanilla extract
- A pinch sea salt
- ½ cup sugar
- 3 tbsp. cornstarch

Directions:

1. In a medium saucepan, combine 2 cups of milk with the vanilla, salt, and sugar. Bring to a boil over medium-high heat, stirring constantly.
2. In a small bowl, whisk together the cornstarch and the remaining ¼ cup of milk.
3. Whisking constantly, pour the cornstarch mixture into the boiling milk mixture. Boil for 1 minute. Reduce the heat to low and simmer, stirring until thick.
4. Refrigerate for 6 hours before serving.

Nutrition:

- Calories: 112
- Fats: <1 g
- Sodium: 52 mg
- Carbs: 25 g
- Fiber: 0 g
- Protein: 3 g

2.   Maple-Ginger Pudding

Preparation Time: 5 minutes
Cooking Time: 10 minutes
Servings: 86
Ingredients:

- 2 ¼ cups nonfat milk, divided
- 1 tbsp. fresh ginger, grated
- ½ cup pure maple syrup
- ½ tsp. orange zest, grated
- 3 tbsp. cornstarch

Directions:

1. In a medium saucepan, combine 2 cups of milk with the ginger, maple syrup, and orange zest. Bring to a boil over medium-high heat, stirring constantly.
2. In a small bowl, whisk together the cornstarch and the remaining ¼ cup of milk.
3. Whisking constantly, pour the cornstarch mixture into the boiling milk mixture. Boil for 1 minute. Reduce the heat to low and simmer, stirring, until thick.
4. Refrigerate for 6 hours before serving.

Nutrition:

- Calories: 116
- Fats: <1 g
- Sodium: 41 mg
- Carbs: 26 g
- Fiber: 0 g
- Protein: 3 g

3.   Pumpkin-Maple Custard

Preparation Time: 5 minutes
Cooking Time: 10 minutes
Servings: 6
Ingredients:

- 1 ¾ cups nonfat milk, divided
- 1 tbsp. fresh ginger, grated
- ½ cup pure maple syrup
- ½ cup pumpkin puree (not pumpkin pie filling)
- 3 tbsp. cornstarch

Directions:

1. In a medium saucepan, combine 1 ½ cups of milk with the ginger, maple syrup, and pumpkin puree. Bring to a boil over medium-high heat, whisking constantly.
2. In a small bowl, whisk together the cornstarch and the remaining ¼ cup of milk.
3. Whisking constantly, pour the cornstarch mixture into the boiling milk mixture. Boil for 1 minute. Reduce the heat to low and simmer, stirring, until thick.
4. Refrigerate for 6 hours before serving.

Nutrition:

- Calories: 115
- Fats: <1 g
- Sodium: 33 mg
- Carbs: 26 g
- Fiber: 1 g
- Protein: 3 g

4.   Gingered Red Applesauce

Preparation Time: 5 minutes
Cooking Time: 15 minutes
Servings: 4
Ingredients:

- 4 red apples, peeled, cored, and chopped
- ¼ cup water
- 2 tbsp. fresh ginger, grated
- 1 tsp. cinnamon

Directions:

1. In a large pot, bring the apples, water, ginger, and cinnamon to a boil over medium-high heat, stirring occasionally.
2. Boil uncovered and stirring occasionally, until the apples are soft, about 10 minutes.
3. Turn off the heat and let cool.
4. Transfer the mixture to a blender or food processor and blend until smooth.

Nutrition:

- Calories: 76 Fats: <1 g
- Sodium: 1 mg Carbs: 20 g
- Fiber: 4 g Protein: <1 g

5.   Ginger-Berry Yogurt Pops

Preparation Time: 30 minutes
Cooking Time: 0 minutes
Servings: 4
Ingredients:

- 2 cups fresh berries
- 2 cups plain nonfat yogurt
- 2 tbsp. honey
- 1 tbsp. fresh ginger, grated

Directions:

1. In a blender or food processor, combine all the ingredients. Blend until smooth.
2. Pour the mixture into molds or cups and freeze until solid, about 6 hours.

Nutrition:

- Calories: 117
- Fats: <1 g
- Sodium: 81 mg
- Carbs: 24 g
- Fiber: 4 g
- Protein: 7 g

6.   Bananas with Maple Brown Sugar Sauce

Preparation Time: 5 minutes
Cooking Time: 10 minutes
Servings: 4
Ingredients:

- 2 tbsp. neutral-flavored oil or coconut oil
- 2 bananas, peeled and split in half lengthwise, then halved crosswise
- ¼ cup pure maple syrup
- ¼ cup brown sugar
- ½ tsp. cinnamon

Directions:

1. Place a large nonstick skillet over medium-high heat and add the oil. Once hot, add the bananas in a single layer and cook until browned on both sides, about 5 minutes.
2. Add the maple syrup, brown sugar, and cinnamon. Cook while stirring occasionally until the brown sugar dissolves. Serve warm.

Nutrition:

- Calories: 199
- Fats: 7 g
- Sodium: 6 mg
- Carbs: 39 g
- Fiber: 2 g
- Protein: 1 g

7.   Honey-Cinnamon   Poached Pears

Preparation Time: 5 minutes
Cooking Time: 40 minutes
Servings: 4
Ingredients:

- 2 cups pear juice
- 3 tbsp. honey
- 2 cinnamon sticks
- 4 pears, peeled

Directions:

1. In a large pot, bring the pear juice, honey, and cinnamon sticks to a boil over medium-high heat.
2. Add the pears and bring to a simmer. Reduce the heat to medium-low.
3. Cover and simmer until the pears are tender, about 20 minutes. Remove the pears from the liquid and set aside.
4. Bring the liquid to a boil over medium-high heat. Cook uncovered while stirring occasionally, until the liquid is syrupy, about 10 minutes. Discard the cinnamon sticks.
5. Serve the pears warm with the syrup spooned over the top.

Flavor Boost: Add 3 cardamom pods to the poaching liquid along with one 1-inch piece of ginger.
Nutrition:

- Calories: 185
- Fats: <1 g
- Sodium: 6 mg
- Carbs: 48 g
- Fiber: 5 g
- Protein: 1 g

8.   Baked Red Apples

Preparation Time: 5 minutes
Cooking Time: 50 minutes
Servings: 4
Ingredients:

- 4 red apples, tops cut off and cored
- ¼ cup brown sugar
- 1 tsp. cinnamon
- 1 tsp. ground ginger
- 4 tbsp. pure maple syrup

Directions:

1. Preheat the oven to 375°F.
2. Place the apples cut-side up on a 9-inch square baking pan.
3. In a small bowl, mix the brown sugar, cinnamon, and ginger.
4. Spoon the mixture into the hollow core of the apples.
5. Pour 1 tablespoon of syrup over each of the apples.
6. Bake until the apples are soft, about 40 to 50 minutes.
7. Serve hot.

Flavor Boost: Crumble 1 graham cracker over the top of each of the baked apples and serve them with nonfat frozen vanilla yogurt.
Nutrition:

- Calories: 161
- Fats: <1 g
- Sodium: 6 mg
- Carbs: 45 g
- Fiber: 4 g
- Protein: <1 g

9. Froyo with Blueberry Sauce

Preparation Time: 5 minutes
Cooking Time: 10 minutes
Servings: 4
Ingredients:

- 2 cups fresh blueberries
- ½ cup sugar
- ½ tsp. orange zest, grated
- ¼ cup water
- 4 scoops fat-free, frozen vanilla yogurt

Directions:

1. In a medium saucepan, bring the blueberries, sugar, orange zest, and water to a boil over medium-high heat, stirring often.
2. Reduce the heat to medium-low. Simmer while smashing the blueberries as you do until the sauce thickens, about 5 minutes.
3. Cool slightly and then serve over the frozen yogurt.

Nutrition:

- Calories: 226
- Fats: 0 g
- Sodium: 54 mg
- Carbs: 55 g
- Fiber: 2 g
- Protein: 4 g

10. Flourless Peanut Butter Cookies

Preparation Time: 5 minutes
Cooking Time: 10 minutes
Servings: 15
Ingredients:

- 1 cup creamy peanut butter (or almond or cashew butter)
- 1 cup brown sugar
- 1 large egg, beaten
- ½ tsp. vanilla extract

Directions:

1. Preheat the oven to 350°F. Line a baking sheet with parchment paper.
2. In a medium bowl or mixer, cream together all the ingredients.
3. Drop 1-tbsp. portions of the batter on the prepared baking sheet. Use a fork to flatten the tops.
4. Bake until golden, about 8 to 10 minutes.
5. Let cool for 2 minutes, then transfer to a wire rack to cool completely.

Flavor Boost: Add texture by stirring in ¼ cup of chopped peanuts to the batter. You can also create a thumbprint in the middle of the cookie instead of flattening it with a fork, and spoon in ½ teaspoon of jam.

Nutrition:

- Calories: 143
- Fats: 9 g
- Sodium: 88 mg
- Carbs: 16 g
- Fiber: 1 g
- Protein: 5 g

11. Mixed Berry Popsicles

Preparation Time: 1 hour
Cooking Time: 10 hours
Servings: 10
Ingredients:

- 1 cup blackberries
- 1 cup boysenberries
- 1 cup strawberries
- 1 cup raspberries
- 4 tbsp. honey
- 4 tsp. lemon juice

Directions:

1. In your food processor, put the blackberries. Add 1 tablespoon of honey and 1 teaspoon of lemon juice. Pulse until a fine puree is available to you.
2. In your popsicle molds, pour the blackberry puree into the rim. Place it for 15 minutes in the freezer.
3. When your popsicle mold is in the fridge, wash your food processor.
4. Boysenberries, then raspberries, and then strawberries. Repeat the first two stages.
5. In the popsicle mold, put the popsicle sticks and place them in the freezer for at least 4 hours to harden fully.

Nutrition:

- Calories: 49 Carbs: 12 g
- Potassium: 86 mg Fiber: 2 g
- Sugar: 9 g Vitamin A: 40 mg
- Vitamin C: 15.8 mg Calcium: 13 mg
- Iron: 0.4 mg

12. Chocolate Avocado Pudding

Preparation Time: 40 minutes
Cooking Time: 0 minutes
Servings: 4
Ingredients:

- 2 large avocados, peeled, pitted, and cubed
- ½ cup unsweetened cocoa powder
- ½ cup brown sugar
- ⅓ cup coconut milk
- 2 tsp. vanilla extract
- A pinch ground cinnamon

Directions:

1. In a blender, mix the avocado, cocoa powder, brown sugar, coconut milk, vanilla extract, and cinnamon until soft. Refrigerate the pudding for about 30 minutes until it is ready.

Nutrition:

- Calories: 400 Protein: 5.4 g
- Carbs: 45.9 g Fats: 26.3 g Sodium: 22.6 mg

13. Instant Frozen Berry Yogurt

Preparation Time: 1 minute
Cooking Time: 0 minutes
Servings: 4
Ingredients:

- 8 ¾ oz. frozen mixed berry
- 8 ¾ oz. Greek yogurt
- 1 tbsp. honey

Directions:

1. In a food processor, mix the berries, yogurt, and honey or agave syrup for 20 seconds, or until the ice cream texture is smooth. Scoop and serve in bowls.

Nutrition:

- Calories: 70
- Fats: 0 g
- Carbs: 10 g
- Sugar: 10 g
- Fiber: 2 g
- Protein: 7 g
- Salt: 0.1 g

14. Chocolate Protein Balls

Preparation Time: 40 minutes
Cooking Time: 0 minutes
Servings: 10
Ingredients:

- 1 cup rolled oats
- ½ cup natural peanut butter
- ⅓ cup honey
- ¼ cup dark chocolate, chopped
- 2 tbsp. flax seeds
- 2 tbsp. chia seeds
- 1 tbsp. chocolate-flavored protein powder, or as needed

Directions:

1. In a bowl, whisk together the oats, peanut butter, honey, chocolate, flax seeds, chia seeds, and protein powder until mixed evenly. Cover the plastic wrap with a bowl and refrigerate for 30 minutes.
2. Scoop the balls into a chilled mixture. Keep it cold before you serve.

Nutrition:

- Calories: 188
- Protein: 5.8 g
- Carbs: 21.5 g
- Fats: 9.9 g
- Cholesterol: 0.2 mg
- Sodium: 67.5 mg

15.   Mozzarella Balls Recipe

Preparation Time: 10 minutes
Cooking Time: 5 minutes
Servings: 8
Ingredients:

- 1 package string cheese
- 2 cups panko bread crumbs
- 2 tsp. Italian seasoning
- 1 tsp. parsley
- 1 cup milk
- 1 cup flour
- Marinara Sauce, for serving (homemade or store-bought)
- Oil, for frying

Directions:

1. Split the cheese into 1-inch pieces.
2. In a bowl, by pouring the milk and setting it aside, prepare the coating form. Put 1 cup of flour in a plastic bag and add 2 cups of panko mixed with seasonings into another bag.
3. Place the cheese one handful at a time in the milk.
4. Toss it in the bag of flour and shake well.
5. Put the cheese back in the bowl of milk, and then coat it well.
6. Toss and shake in the panko bag until uniformly covered.
7. Place the bites of mozzarella on a plate or in a bag, and freeze for a minimum of 2 hours.
8. Heat the oil on medium heat. Fry until golden brown in hot oil. Be sure to take them out of the oil until they get too hot; otherwise, from the breading, the cheese will ooze.
9. Serve soft with marinara sauce. Enjoy!

Nutrition:

- Fats: 1 g
- Cholesterol: 3 mg
- Sodium: 124 mg
- Potassium: 92 mg
- Carbs: 24 g
- Fiber: 1 g
- Sugar: 2 g
- Protein: 4 g

16.   Strawberry Frozen Yogurt

Preparation Time: 5 minutes
Cooking Time: 4 hours
Servings: 4
Ingredients:

- 2 tbsp. honey
- 1 cup low-fat, plain Greek yogurt
- 4 cups frozen strawberries
- 2 tsp. vanilla extract
- 1 tsp. lemon juice, freshly squeezed

Directions:

1. In a food processor combine the yogurt, strawberries, honey, vanilla, and lemon juice. Pulse until crumbly, then process until the mixture becomes creamy. Transfer to a standard-size loaf pan. Cover and freeze for 2 hours, or until frozen but still soft enough to scoop it into servings.

Ingredient Tip: Berries are a great source of fiber and antioxidants and a wonderful addition to your diet. Switch it up and try this recipe with raspberries, blueberries, cranberries, or whatever you find in season and available.

Nutrition:

- Calories: 135
- Fats: 1 g
- Protein: 6 g
- Carbs: 25 g
- Fiber: 3 g
- Sugar: 17 g
- Sodium: 39 mg

17. Chocolate Protein Pudding Pops

Preparation Time: 5 minutes
Cooking Time: 10 minutes
Servings: 4
Ingredients:

- 1 (4-oz.) package chocolate-flavored instant pudding
- 2 cups cold low-fat milk
- 2 scoops chocolate protein powder

Directions:

1. In a medium bowl, whisk the pudding mix, milk, and protein powder for at least 2 min.
2. Spoon into ice pop molds or paper cups. Insert an ice pop stick into the center of each mold or cup.
3. Freeze for 4 hours, or until firm. Remove from the molds or cups before servings.

Nutrition:

- Calories: 215
- Fats: 2 g
- Protein: 12 g
- Carbs: 36 g
- Fiber: 0 g
- Sugar: 27 g
- Sodium: 480 mg

18. Red Energy Wonders

Preparation Time: 15 minutes
Cooking Time: 15 minutes
Servings: 5–6
Ingredients:

- 5 tbsp. almond butter
- 2 ⅓ cups coconut, shredded and divided into a 225 ml portion and a 100 ml portion
- ½ cup oats, rolled
- ½ cup strawberries
- ½ cup pitiless almonds, dates, and Medrol

Directions:

1. Place the 225-ml portion of coconut and all the rest of the ingredients in a food processor. At high speed, process until smooth and fully mixed.
2. Pour the remaining coconut onto a plate. With a spoon, scoop out 1 tablespoon of the mixture and form it into a ball. Roll this ball around in the coconut, then place it on a plate lined with parchment paper. Repeat until all of the mixture is used.
3. Place the plate in the fridge for at least 2 hours before servings. Keep energy wonders in an air-tight container in the fridge.

Nutrition:

- Calories: 191
- Carbs: 17.9 g
- Protein: 6.3 g
- Fats: 12 g
- Saturated Fat: 5.4 g
- Cholesterol: 7 mg
- Sodium: 101 mg
- Fiber: 2.8 g
- Sugar: 8.6 g

19. Bella's Apple Crisp

Preparation Time: 20 minutes
Cooking Time: 20 minutes
Servings: 4
Ingredients:

- 4 apples, hard and crisp, cored and sliced
- ½ lemon
- 2 tbsp. water
- 2 tbsp. agave nectar (or 1 tbsp. honey)
- 2 tbsp Syrup

For Toppings:

- ¾ cup plus 1 tbsp. and 1 tsp. old-fashioned rolled oats
- 2 tbsp. butter, cold
- ½ tsp. cinnamon
- ½ cup walnuts, chopped
- Fat-free, sugar-free ice cream, for serving (optional)

Directions:

1. Heat oven to 350ºF.
2. Place the sliced apples in the bottom of an 8-inch pie plate or square cake pan.
3. Drizzle the water, lemon juice, and syrup over the apples.
4. In a mixing bowl, stir together the oats and cinnamon. Use a pastry cutter or 2 knives to cut in the butter mixture until it resembles coarse breadcrumbs.
5. Stir in the chopped nuts.
6. Sprinkle the mixture over the apples, covering them completely.
7. Cover the pan with tin foil and slide it into the middle of the oven for 20 minutes.
8. Remove tin foil from the pan and continue to bake for another 10 to 15 minutes, or until the topping is golden brown. (It can be with a dab of fat-free, sugar-free ice cream.)

Nutrition:

- Calories: 424
- Carbs: 74.3 g
- Protein: 14.6 g
- Fats: 9.4 g
- Cholesterol: 94 mg
- Sodium: 572 mg
- Fiber: 11.3 g
- Sugar: 24.2 g

20. Chocolate Almond Ginger Mousse

Preparation Time: 10 minutes
Cooking Time: 30 minutes (plus 4 hours of cooling time)
Servings: 4
Ingredients:

- 1 ⅓ cup plus 1 tsp. milk, skim, and cold
- 1 instant pudding package, fat-free and sugar-free
- ¼ tsp. ginger, dried
- 1 tbsp. almonds, sliced

Directions:

1. Pour the cold milk into a mixing bowl. Beating steadily with a wire whisk, add the pudding mix and dried ginger. Keep whisking for 2 minutes. Fold in the cool whip topping.
2. Spoon it into 5 pudding cups and refrigerate them until needed. Garnish with the sliced almonds just before serving.

Nutrition:

- Calories: 310
- Carbs: 21 g
- Protein: 3.9 g
- Fats: 26.4 g
- Saturated Fat: 9.5 g
- PolyunSaturated Fat: 16.9 g
- Sodium: 90 mg
- Fiber: 10.2 g
- Sugar: 7.1 g

21.   Peanut Butter Joy Cookies

Preparation Time: 30 minutes
Cooking Time: 45 minutes
Servings: 3–4
Ingredients:

- 1 cup plus 2 tsp. quick oats
- 1 cup plus 2 tsp. peanut butter, unsweetened
- 1 cup plus 2 tsp. Splenda®
- 1 tsp. vanilla
- ½ tsp. dried cinnamon
- 1 egg

Directions:

1. Preheat the oven to 350°F.
2. Place the peanut butter and Splenda® in a mixing bowl. Using a sturdy spoon or hand beater, beat the two together until smooth. Add in the egg, keep mixing, and then add the vanilla.
3. Last, add in the oats and cinnamon. Continue to mix until it is nice, smooth dough.
4. Scoop the dough out with the help of a dessert spoon, and using your hands, roll it into balls. Place the balls on a cookie sheet and squish them gently down with a fork.
5. Place the cookies in the oven for 8 minutes, or until golden brown. Wait for them to cool before lifting off the pan.

Nutrition:

- Calories: 338
- Protein: 2.5 g
- Carbs: 10.8 g
- Dietary Fibers: 7.9 g
- Fats: 34.1 g

22.   Broccoli Cauliflower Puree

Preparation Time: 15 minutes
Cooking Time: 20 minutes
Servings: 2
Ingredients:

- 2 cups fresh broccoli chopped
- 2 cups fresh cauliflower, chopped
- ½ cup skim milk
- ½ tsp. salt
- ½ tsp. Italian seasoning
- ¼ tsp. cumin, ground
- 1 tbsp. fresh parsley, finely chopped
- 1 tbsp. olive oil
- 1 tsp. dry mint, ground

Directions:

1. Wash and roughly chop the cauliflower. Place it in a deep pot and add a pinch of salt. Cook for about 15–20 minutes. When done, drain and transfer it to a food processor. Set aside.
2. Wash the broccoli and chop it into bite-sized pieces. Add it to the food processor along with milk, salt, Italian seasoning, cumin, parsley, and mint. Gradually add olive oil and blend until nicely pureed.
3. Serve with some fresh carrots and celery.

Nutrition:

- Calories: 138
- Protein: 6.1 g
- Carbs: 12.7 g
- Dietary Fibers: 4.6 g
- Fats: 7.5 g

23. Grilled Avocado in Curry Sauce

Preparation Time: 15 minutes
Cooking Time: 8 minutes
Servings: 2
Ingredients:

- 1 large avocado, chopped
- ¼ cup water
- 1 tbsp. curry, ground
- 2 tbsp. olive oil
- 1 tsp. soy sauce
- 1 tsp. fresh parsley, finely chopped
- ¼ tsp. red pepper flakes
- ¼ tsp. sea salt

Directions:

1. Peel the avocado and cut it lengthwise in half. Remove the pit and cut the remaining avocado into small chunks. Set aside.
2. Heat the olive oil in a large saucepan over a medium-high temperature.
3. In a small bowl, combine the ground curry, soy sauce, parsley, red pepper, and sea salt. Add the water and cook for about 5 minutes, stirring occasionally.
4. Add the chopped avocado, stir well, and cook for 3 more minutes, or until all the liquid evaporates. Turn off the heat and cover. Let it stand for about 15–20 minutes before serving.

Nutrition:

- Calories: 338
- Protein: 2.5 g
- Carbs: 10.8 g
- Dietary Fibers: 7.9 g
- Fats: 34.1 g

24. Sweet Pumpkin Pudding

Preparation Time: 15 minutes
Cooking Time: 15 minutes
Servings: 4
Ingredients:

- 1 lb. pumpkin, peeled and chopped into bite-sized pieces
- 2 tbsp. honey
- ½ cup cornstarch
- 4 cups pumpkin juice, unsweetened
- 1 tsp. cinnamon, ground
- 3 cloves, freshly ground
- 2 cups Orange juice

Directions:

1. Peel and prepare the pumpkin. Scrape out seeds and chop them into bite-sized pieces. Set aside.
2. In a small bowl, combine the pumpkin juice, honey, orange juice, cinnamon, and cornstarch.
3. Place the pumpkin chops in a large pot and pour the pumpkin juice mixture. Stir well and then finally add the cloves. Stir until well incorporated and heat up until almost boiling. Reduce the heat to low and cook for about 15 minutes, or until the mixture thickens.
4. Remove from the heat and transfer them to the bowls immediately. Set aside to cool completely and then refrigerate for 15 minutes before serving, or simply chill overnight.

Nutrition:

- Calories: 232
- Protein: 2.7 g
- Carbs: 56 g
- Dietary Fibers: 4.6 g
- Fats: 0.9 g

25.   Avocado Detox Smoothie

Preparation Time: 10 minutes
Cooking Time: 30 minutes
Servings: 2
Ingredients:

- ½ avocado, peeled and roughly chopped
- 1 banana, peeled and chopped
- A handful baby spinach, torn
- 1 tbsp. powdered stevia
- 1 tsp. ground turmeric
- 1 tbsp. ground flaxseed
- 1 tbsp. goji berries

Directions:

1. Peel the avocado and cut it in half. Remove the pit and chop one half into small pieces. Wrap the other half in plastic foil and refrigerate it for later.
2. Peel the banana and cut it into thin slices. Set aside.
3. Rinse the spinach thoroughly under cold running water using a colander. Chop it into small pieces and set aside.
4. Now combine the avocado, banana, spinach, turmeric, flaxseed, and goji berries in a blender. Process until well combined.
5. Transfer to a serving glass and add few ice cubes.
6. Serve immediately.

Nutrition:

- Calories: 221 Protein: 3.1 g
- Carbs: 28.6 g Dietary Fibers: 7.5 g
- Fats: 11.8 g

26.   Avocado Hummus

Preparation Time: 15 minutes
Cooking Time: 0 minutes
Servings: 2
Ingredients:

- 1 cup edamame
- ½ avocado, chopped
- 1 tbsp. lemon juice
- 2 tbsp. olive oil
- ½ tsp. minced garlic
- ½ tsp. onion powder
- 1 tsp. tahini

Directions:

1. Add all of these ingredients into a blender and blend until smooth. Serve with some vegetables and enjoy it.

Nutrition:

- Calories: 112 Fats: 4 g
- Carbs: 18 g Protein: 7 g
- Sodium: 126 mg

27.   Raspberry Sorbet

Preparation Time: 10 minutes
Cooking Time: 0 minutes
Servings: 2
Ingredients:

- 1 tbsp. honey
- ¼ cup coconut water
- 12 oz. raspberries

Directions:

1. We need to take all of those ingredients that we listed above and add them inside a prepared blender. Blend until it is nice and smooth.
2. Pour this into a container and add the lid to the top. Add to the freezer to set for a few hours before serving.

Nutrition:

- Calories: 131
- Fats: 4 g
- Carbs: 8 g
- Protein: 6 g
- Sodium: 212 mg

28.   Tomato,   Basil,   and Cucumber Salad

Preparation Time: 15 minutes
Cooking Time: 0 minutes
Servings: 6
Ingredients:

- 1 large cucumber, seeded and sliced
- 4 medium tomatoes, quartered
- 1 medium red onion, thinly sliced
- ½ cup fresh basil, chopped
- 3 tbsp. red wine vinegar
- 1 tbsp. extra-virgin olive oil
- ½ tsp. Dijon mustard
- ½ tsp. black pepper, freshly ground

Directions:

1. In a medium bowl, mix the cucumber, tomatoes, red onion, and basil.
2. In a small bowl, whisk together the vinegar, olive oil, mustard, and pepper.
3. Pour the dressing over the vegetables, and gently stir until well combined.
4. Cover and chill for at least 30 minutes before serving.

Nutrition:

- Calories: 72 Fats: 4 g
- Protein: 1 g Carbs: 8 g
- Fiber: 1 g Sugar: 4 g
- Sodium: 5 mg

29.   Mashed Cauliflower

Preparation Time: 10 minutes
Cooking Time: 5 minutes
Servings: 4
Ingredients:

- 1 large cauliflower head
- ¼ cup water
- ⅓ cup low-fat buttermilk
- 1 tbsp. minced garlic
- 1 tbsp. extra-virgin olive oil

Directions:

1. Break the cauliflower into small florets. Place them in a large microwave-safe bowl with the water. Cover and microwave for about 5 minutes, or until the cauliflower is soft. Drain the water from the bowl.
2. Using a food processor, purée the buttermilk, cauliflower, garlic, and olive oil on medium speed until the cauliflower is smooth and creamy.
3. Serve immediately.

Ingredient Tip: You can buy buttermilk in most supermarkets, but it's just as easy to make your own. Mix 1 teaspoon of freshly squeezed lemon juice with ⅓ cup of low-fat milk. Let the mixture sit for about 10 minutes, or until the milk begins to thicken.

Cooking Tip: For even more flavor, microwave the cauliflower with the chicken or vegetable broth instead of water, and add ½ cup of shredded Parmigiano-Reggiano cheese when you purée the mixture. You can add protein to this dish by blending in powdered egg whites or unflavored protein powder after the first purée (puree until smooth and creamy, and then add the protein powder and purée to incorporate).

Nutrition:

- Calories: 62
- Fats: 2 g
- Protein: 3 g
- Carbs: 8 g
- Fiber: 3 g
- Sugar: 3 g
- Sodium: 54 mg

30.   Low Acid Raspberry Cobbler

Preparation Time: 90 minutes
Cooking Time: 12 minutes
Servings: 8
Ingredients:

- 1 cup granulated sugar
- 2 cups all-purpose flour
- ½ tsp. salt
- 2 ½ tsp. baking powder
- ⅔ cup milk
- 3 tbsp. unsalted butter, melted
- 1 large egg, lightly beaten
- 1 tsp. vanilla extract
- 2 cups raspberries
- Vanilla ice cream (optional)

Directions:

1. Preheat the oven to 350°F. Prepare a square baking pan by spraying the bottom and sides with cooking oil. Set the pan to the side for the moment.
2. In a large mixing bowl, stir together the sugar, flour, salt, and baking powder. Mix in the melted butter, vanilla, milk, and beaten egg until well combined.
3. Fold in the raspberries.
4. Pour the batter into the prepared pan. Place the pan in the oven and bake for about 45 minutes. (The top of the cobbler should be firm and tight.)
5. Let the cobbler cool a bit before serving. If desired, add a scoop of vanilla ice cream to the top or side of the cobbler.

Nutrition:

- Fats: 6 g
- Saturated Fat: 1 g
- Sodium: 37 mg
- Potassium: 87 mg
- Fiber: 2 g
- Sugar: 17 g
- Vitamin A: 130IU
- Vitamin C: 31 mg
- Calcium: 23 mg
- Iron: 1 mg

31. I Can't Believe It's Not Fudge

Preparation Time: 150 minutes
Cooking Time: 12 minutes
Servings: 10
Ingredients:

- 1 cup dates, pitted
- 2 cups cashews, soaked and drained
- 2 tbsp. carob powder
- 1 cup raisins
- 1 cup walnuts, chopped
- 1 cup flaxseed meal
- ½ cup water, distilled
- ½ cup pineapple juice

Directions:

1. Blend the dates, carob powder, cashews, raisins, walnuts, and pineapple juice in a blender or food processor. Continue blending until smooth.
2. Stir in the water and flaxseed meal until well combined.
3. Press the mixture into a baking sheet. Place the sheet in the freezer for about 2 hours. Cut the fudge into squares before serving.

Nutrition:

- Calories: 165
- Carbs: 28 g
- Protein: 1 g

32. Low-Acid Almond Meringues

Preparation Time: 140 minutes
Cooking Time: 60 minutes
Servings: 3
Ingredients:

- 3 large egg whites
- ¾ cup granulated sugar
- ⅓ cup sliced almonds, toasted and crushed

Directions:

1. Preheat the oven to 225°F.
2. Beat the egg whites and salt until peaks begin to form. Continue to beat while adding the granulated sugar.
3. Line a baking sheet with parchment paper.
4. Transfer the meringues into a pastry bag. Use the pastry bag to pipe the meringues directly onto the parchment paper in a lattice style. Sprinkle the almonds directly on top.
5. Place the baking sheet in the preheated oven and bake for about 60 minutes. You want the meringues to be a golden pale color with a crispy texture.
6. Remove the baking sheet from the oven and let the meringues cool for about an hour before serving.

Nutrition:

- Calories: 456
- Carbs: 27 g
- Protein: 14 g
- Fats: 26 g
- Saturated Fat: 2 g
- Cholesterol: 9 mg

33. Low Acid Angel Food Cake

Preparation Time: 75 minutes
Cooking Time: 35 minutes
Servings: 8
Ingredients:

- 1 cup granulated sugar
- 1 cup cake flour, sifted
- 1 tsp. cream of tartar
- ½ tsp. salt
- 12 large egg whites, room temperature
- 2 tsp. vanilla

Directions:

1. Preheat the oven to 375ºF.
2. Whisk together the flour and ¾ cup of sugar.
3. In a second bowl, beat the egg whites until they are thick. Stir in the salt, cream of tartar, and vanilla. Continue to beat until stiff peaks begin to form. Stir in the remaining ¼ cup of sugar.
4. Combine the flour mixture with the egg mixture until well mixed. Pour this mixture into a nonstick tube pan. Place the pan in the oven and bake for about 30 to 35 minutes.
5. Remove the pan from the oven and let cool before serving.

Nutrition:

- Fats: 11 g
- Saturated Fat: 1 g
- Sodium: 1 mg
- Potassium: 37 mg
- Fiber: 1 g
- Sugar: 1 g

34. Pound Cake

Preparation Time: 75 minutes
Cooking Time: 1 hour (plus more)
Servings: 8
Ingredients:

- 2 cups all-purpose flour
- ¼ tsp. salt
- 1 tbsp. baking powder
- 1 ½ cups granulated sugar
- ½ cup unsalted butter, softened
- 4 large egg whites, lightly beaten
- 2 tsp. vanilla extract
- 1 ½ cups fat-free sour cream
- Powdered sugar, for serving

Directions:

1. Preheat your oven to 350ºF. Prepare a Bundt® pan by spraying the bottom and sides with cooking oil. Set the pan to the side for the moment.
2. In a small bowl, mix the flour, salt, and baking soda. Set it aside for now.
3. In a large mixing bowl, cream the butter and sugar together. Stir in the egg whites, vanilla, and sour cream. Continue stirring until well mixed.
4. Gradually stir the flour mixture into the butter mixture until combined but not overmixed.
5. Transfer the batter into the prepared Bundt® pan from step 1. Place the pan in the oven and let bake for about 1 hour. The pound cake is done when a toothpick inserted in the middle comes out clean.
6. Remove the pan from the oven and let cool completely before turning the cake out of the pan. Dust with powdered sugar before serving.

Nutrition:

- Potassium: 106 mg
- Fiber: 3 g
- Sugar: 6 g
- Vitamin A: 13IU
- Vitamin C: 1 mg
- Calcium: 54 mg
- Iron: 1 mg

35. Blueberry Cherry Crisp

Preparation Time: 5 minutes
Cooking Time: 38 minutes
Servings: 8
Ingredients:

- 1 cup old-fashioned oatmeal
- ⅓ cup coconut flour
- ½ cup macadamia nuts, chopped
- 2 tbsp. coconut oil
- 3 tbsp. almond butter
- 2 tbsp. honey
- 1 tsp. cinnamon
- ¼ tsp. nutmeg
- ⅛ tsp. sea salt
- 4 cups frozen cherries, thawed
- 2 cups frozen blueberries

Directions:

1. Set the oven to 375°F. Add the almond butter to a 9x9-inch glass dish.
2. Mix the oatmeal with nuts and flours in a glass bowl.
3. Heat the honey with the almond butter, coconut oil, nutmeg, sea salt, and cinnamon in a pan.
4. Cook for 3 minutes on low heat while stirring.
5. Gradually stir in the oatmeal mixture and keep mixing well.
6. Spread the blueberries and cherries in the glass dish.
7. Add the oatmeal mixture to the dish and spread it evenly.
8. Bake for 35 minutes, or until bubbly.
9. Serve.

Nutrition:

- Calories: 252
- Fats: 16 g
- Saturated Fat: 7 g
- Cholesterol: 11 mg
- Sodium: 8 mg
- Carbs: 29 g
- Sugar: 1.8 g
- Fiber: 5 g
- Protein 4 g

36. Baked Apples with Tahini Raisin Filling

Preparation Time: 10 minutes
Cooking Time: 35 minutes
Servings: 4
Ingredients:

- 4 ripe apples, cored
- ¾ cup tahini
- 1 cup apple juice
- 3 tbsp. raisins
- ⅓ cup pecans, chopped
- ¼ tsp. cinnamon
- A dash nutmeg
- A dash vanilla
- ¾ cup boiling water

Directions:

1. Set the oven to 375°F to preheat. Grease a 9x13-inch baking dish with oil.
2. Place the cored apples in the shallow dish.
3. Mix the tahini with ½ cup of apple juice in a small bowl.
4. Stir in the pecans, raisins, nutmeg, vanilla, and cinnamon. Mix well.
5. Stuff this mixture into the core of the apples.
6. Add some boiling water to the baking dish.
7. Pour the remaining apple juice on top.
8. Bake for 35 minutes, or until tender.
9. Serve the apples with the remaining juices on top.

Nutrition:

- Calories: 386
- Fats: 24 g
- Saturated Fat: 3 g
- Cholesterol: 0 mg
- Sodium: 19 mg
- Carbs: 41 g
- Sugar: 1.9 g
- Fiber: 7 g
- Protein: 8 g

37.   Coconut Rice Pudding

Preparation Time: 5 minutes
Cooking Time: 10 minutes
Servings: 4
Ingredients:

- ¾ cup low-fat milk
- ½ cup coconut milk
- 1 large pear, grated
- 2 tbsp. honey
- ¼ cup dried cranberries
- 1 (1-oz.) package fat-free, sugar-free vanilla pudding mix
- 2 cups cooked brown rice
- ¼ cup shredded coconut
- ½ tsp. ground ginger

Directions:

1. Cook the grated pears with the milk, coconut milk, and honey in a pan over medium heat.
2. Boil the mixture, then remove it from the heat.
3. Gradually stir in the pudding mix, coconut, ginger, and rice.
4. Mix well and let this mixture sit for 10 minutes.
5. Stir in the cranberries and mix gently.
6. Serve.

Nutrition:

- Calories: 190
- Fats: 6 g
- Saturated Fat: 2 g
- Cholesterol: 2 mg
- Sodium: 244 mg
- Carbs: 31 g
- Sugar: 3.6 g
- Fiber: 0.8 g
- Protein: 3 g

38.   Peach Cobbler

Preparation Time: 10 minutes
Cooking Time: 30 minutes
Servings: 6
Ingredients:

- ½ tsp. ground cinnamon
- 1 tbsp. vanilla extract
- 2 tbsp. xanthan gum
- ¼ cup peach juice
- 1 cup peach nectar
- ¾–1 lb. fresh peaches, sliced
- 1 tbsp. margarine
- 1 cup dry pancake mix
- ⅔ cup coconut flour
- ½ cup Splenda®
- ⅔ cup evaporated skim milk

For the Topping:

- ½ tsp. nutmeg and 1 tbsp. Splenda®

Directions:

1. Whisk the vanilla with peach, nectar, peach juice, xanthan gum, and cinnamon in a pan.
2. Cook well until it bubbles and thickens.
3. Stir in the sliced peaches and reduce the heat. Let it simmer for 10 minutes.
4. Heat the margarine in a saucepan and keep it aside.
5. Grease an 8-inch square dish with cooking oil and add it to the peach mixture.
6. Mix the melted margarine with the Splenda®, flour, pancake mix, and milk in a separate bowl.
7. Pour this mixture over the peach mixture.
8. Sprinkle Splenda® and nutmeg over it.
9. Bake at 400°F for about 20 minutes, or until golden brown.
10. Slice and serve.

Nutrition:

- Calories: 271
- Fats: 4 g
- Saturated Fat: 1 g
- Cholesterol: 0 mg
- Sodium: 263 mg
- Carbs: 9.6 g
- Sugar: 0.1 g
- Fiber: 3.8 g
- Protein: 7.6 g

39.   Vanilla Parfait

Preparation Time: 10 minutes
Cooking Time: 0 minutes
Servings: 2
Ingredients:

- 1 cup unsweetened vanilla milk
- 1 cup plain, low-fat Greek yogurt
- 2 tbsp. agaves
- 1 tsp. vanilla
- ⅛ tsp. kosher salt
- ¼ cup chia seeds
- 2 cups strawberries, sliced
- ¼ cup almonds, sliced
- 4 tsp. agaves, for serving

Directions:

1. Mix the milk, yogurt, agave, vanilla, and salt in a medium bowl.
2. Whisk in the chia seeds and let the mixture rest for 25 minutes.
3. Cover the bowl and refrigerate it overnight.
4. Mix the strawberries with the agave and toasted almonds in a bowl.
5. Layer serving glasses with the yogurt pudding and strawberries (alternatively).
6. Serve.

Nutrition:

- Calories: 199
- Fats: 7 g
- Saturated Fat: 3.5 g
- Cholesterol: 125 mg
- Carbs: 7.2 g
- Sugar: 1.4 g
- Fiber: 2.1 g
- Sodium: 135 mg
- Protein: 4.7 g

40.   Pumpkin Pudding Parfaits

Preparation Time: 10 minutes
Cooking Time: 22 minutes
Servings: 6
Ingredients:

- 1 cup pumpkin purée
- ¼ cup packed Splenda®
- ½ tsp. ground cinnamon
- 3 cups almond milk
- 2 tbsp. almond butter
- ½ cup Splenda®
- 3 tbsp. xanthan gum
- 1 tsp. salt
- 4 large egg whites
- 2 tsp. vanilla extract

Directions:

1. Mix the pumpkin purée with the cinnamon and Splenda® in a saucepan.
2. Stir-cook the mixture for 10 minutes, or until smooth.
3. Heat 2 cups of milk with almond butter in a microwave for 2 minutes over high heat.
4. Whisk the Splenda® with the salt and xanthan gum in a large pan.
5. Stir in 1 cup of milk and mix well until smooth.
6. Cook until the mixture thickens.
7. Stir in the vanilla and strain the mixture.
8. Add half of the vanilla pudding to the pumpkin mixture.
9. Mix well and divide the pumpkin pudding into the serving cups.
10. Top the pumpkin pudding with the remaining vanilla pudding.
11. Refrigerate for 4 hours.
12. Garnish as desired and serve.

Nutrition:

- Calories: 151
- Fats: 3.4 g
- Saturated Fat: 7 g
- Cholesterol: 20 mg
- Carbs: 6.4 g
- Sugar: 2.1 g
- Fiber: 4.8 g
- Sodium: 136 mg
- Protein: 4.2 g

41.   Banana Pudding Parfaits

Preparation Time: 10 minutes
Cooking Time: 15 minutes
Servings: 2
Ingredients:

- 1 cup Splenda®
- ¼ cup xanthan gum
- ¼ tsp. salt
- 2 ½ cups almond milk
- 4 large egg whites
- 2 tbsp. unsalted almond butter
- 1 tsp. pure vanilla extract
- 2 bananas, sliced
- 12 shortbread cookies, crumbled

Directions:

1. Mix the Splenda® with the salt, xanthan gum, and milk in a saucepan.
2. Stir-cook until smooth, then whisk in the egg whites.
3. Cook until the mixture bubbles.
4. Strain the mixture and stir in the vanilla and almond butter. Mix well.
5. Layer the serving glasses with the bananas slices, cookies, and pudding.
6. Refrigerate for 1 hour.
7. Serve.

Nutrition:

- Calories: 165
- Fats: 3 g
- Saturated Fat: 0.2 g
- Cholesterol: 09 mg
- Sodium: 7.1 mg
- Carbs: 17.5 g
- Sugar: 1.1 g
- Fiber: 0.5 g
- Protein: 2.2 g

42.   Oatmeal Cookies

Preparation Time: 5 minutes
Cooking Time: 10 minutes
Servings: 6
Ingredients:

- 1 cup coconut flour
- 1 cup quick-cooking oats
- ½ cup Splenda
- ½ tsp. baking powder
- ½ tsp. baking soda
- ½ tsp. salt
- ½ tsp. ground cinnamon
- 2 egg whites
- ⅓ cup corn syrup
- 1 tsp. vanilla extract
- ⅓ cup raisins

Directions:

1. Mix the flour with the oats, baking powder, soda, salt, cinnamon, and Splenda® in a bowl.
2. Fold in the raisins, and mix gently.
3. Drop the batter on the baking sheet spoon by spoon.
4. Bake in the preheated oven at 375°F for 10 minutes.
5. Serve.

Nutrition:

- Calories: 102
- Fats: 1 g
- Saturated Fat: 0 g
- Cholesterol: 0 mg
- Sodium: 138 mg
- Carbs: 24 g
- Fiber: 0 g
- Sugar: 0 g
- Protein: 2

43.   Gingersnaps

Preparation Time: 10 minutes
Cooking Time: 8 minutes
Servings: 6
Ingredients:

- ½ cup unsulphured molasses
- 1 egg white
- 3 ½ cups coconut flour
- 1 tsp. baking soda
- ½ tsp. salt
- 2 tsp. ground ginger
- 1 tsp. cinnamon
- ½ tsp. ground cloves
- ½ tsp. ground nutmeg
- ½ tsp. black pepper, freshly ground

Directions:

1. Whisk the almond butter with Splenda® in a bowl.
2. Stir in the molasses and the egg white. Mix well until smooth.
3. Combine the flour with the salt, spices, and baking soda in a mixing bowl.
4. Stir in the almond butter mixture and mix well at low speed.
5. Divide the dough into halves. Wrap the dough in a plastic sheet.
6. Refrigerate it for 3 hours.
7. Set the oven to 350°F.
8. Unwrap the dough and keep it on a floured surface.
9. Roll the dough into a ⅛-inch-thick sheet.
10. Cut small cookies using a cookie cutter.
11. Set the cookies on a baking sheet lined with parchment paper.
12. Bake for 8 minutes, or until golden brown.
13. Serve.

Nutrition:

- Calories: 209
- Fats: 0.5 g
- Saturated Fat: 11.7 g
- Cholesterol: 58 mg
- Sodium: 163 mg
- Carbs: 19.9 g
- Fiber: 1.5 g
- Sugar: 0.3 g
- Protein: 3.3 g

44.   Coconut Biscotti

Preparation Time: 10 minutes
Cooking Time: 60 minutes
Servings: 6
Ingredients:

- 1 ½ cups coconut flour
- ¾ tsp. baking powder
- ¼ tsp. salt
- ¼ tsp. baking soda
- ⅛ tsp. whole nutmeg, grated
- ¾ cup Splenda®
- 1 tsp. vanilla extract
- 2 egg whites
- 1 cup sweetened coconut, flaked

Directions:

1. Set the oven to 300°F to preheat.
2. Mix all the ingredients in an electric mixer to form a smooth dough.
3. Knead the dough, then make 3-inch rolls out of this dough.
4. Place the rolls on the baking sheet lined with parchment paper.
5. Lightly press each roll and bake at 300°F for 40 minutes.
6. Allow them to cool, then slice the rolls diagonally.
7. Bake for another 20 minutes.
8. Serve.

Nutrition:

- Calories: 237
- Fats: 19.8 g
- Saturated Fat: 1.4 g
- Cholesterol: 10 mg
- Sodium: 719 mg
- Carbs: 55.1 g
- Fiber: 0.9 g
- Sugar: 1.4 g
- Protein: 17.8 g

45. Cheesecake Mousse with Raspberries

Preparation Time: 10 minutes
Cooking Time: 8 minutes
Servings: 6
Ingredients:

- 1 cup light lemonade filling
- 1 (8-oz.) can cream cheese at room temperature
- ¾ cup Splenda® (no-calorie sweetener pellets)
- 1 tbsp. lemon zest
- 1 tbsp. vanilla extract
- 1 cup fresh or frozen raspberries
- Fresh mint, for garnish

Directions:

1. Beat the cream cheese until it is sparkling; add ½ cup of Splenda® granules and mix until melted. Stir in lemon zest and vanilla.
2. Reserve some raspberries for decoration. Crush the rest of the raspberries with a fork and mix them with ¼ cup of Splenda® pellets until they are melted.
3. Lightly add the lump and cheese filling, and then gently but quickly add the crushed raspberries. Divide this mousse into 6 ramekins with a spoon, and keep in the refrigerator until tasting.
4. Garnish the mousses with the reserved raspberries, and garnish with fresh mint before serving.

Nutrition:

- Calories: 259
- Carbs: 37 g
- Protein: 5 g
- Fats: 11 g
- Saturated Fat: 1 g
- Sodium: 197 mg

46. Baked Apples

Preparation Time: 15 minutes
Cooking Time: 18 minutes
Servings: 4
Ingredients:

- 4 apples, cored
- ¼ cup coconut oil, softened
- 4 tsp. ground cinnamon
- ⅛ tsp. ground ginger
- ⅛ tsp. ground nutmeg

Directions:

1. Preheat the oven to 350°F.
2. Fill each apple with 1 tablespoon of coconut oil.
3. Sprinkle each with spices evenly.
4. Arrange the apples on a baking sheet.
5. Bake for about 12–18 minutes.

Nutrition:

- Calories: 240
- Fats: 14.1 g
- Saturated Fat: 11.8 g
- Cholesterol: 0 mg
- Sodium: 2 mg
- Carbs: 32.7 g
- Fiber: 6.6 g
- Sugar: 23.3 g
- Protein: 0.7 g

47.   Berries Granita

Preparation Time: 15 minutes
Cooking Time: 3 hours
Servings: 4
Ingredients:

- ½ cup fresh strawberries, hulled and sliced
- ½ cup fresh raspberries
- ½ cup fresh blueberries
- ½ cup fresh blackberries
- 1 tbsp. pure maple syrup
- 1 tbsp. fresh lemon juice
- 1 cup ice cubes, crushed
- 1 tsp. fresh mint leaves

Directions:

1. In a high-speed blender, add the berries, maple syrup, lemon juice, and ice cubes. Then pulse at high speed until smooth.
2. Transfer the berries mixture evenly into an 8x8-inch baking dish, and freeze for at least 30 minutes.
3. Remove from the freezer and stir the granita completely using a fork.
4. Return it to the freezer and freeze it for about 2–3 hours. Scrape it every 30 minutes with a fork.
5. Place the granita into serving glasses and serve immediately garnished with the mint leaves.

Nutrition:

- Calories: 46
- Fats: 0.3 g
- Saturated Fat: 0 g
- Cholesterol: 0 mg
- Sodium: 4 mg
- Carbs: 11.1 g
- Fiber: 2.8 g
- Sugar: 7.3 g
- Protein: 0.7 g

48.   Pumpkin Ice Cream

Preparation Time: 15 Minutes
Cooking Time: 2 hours and 15 minutes
Servings: 6
Ingredients:

- 15 oz. homemade pumpkin puree
- ½ cup dates, pitted and chopped
- 2 (14-oz.) cans unsweetened coconut milk
- ½ tsp. organic vanilla extract
- 1 ½ tsp. pumpkin pie spice
- ½ tsp. ground cinnamon
- A pinch sea salt

Directions:

1. In a high-speed blender, add all the ingredients and pulse until smooth.
2. Transfer into an air-tight container and freeze for about 1–2 hours.
3. Now transfer the mixture into an ice cream maker and process it according to the manufacturer's instructions.
4. Return the ice cream to the air-tight container and freeze for about 1–2 hours before serving.

Nutrition:

- Calories: 293
- Fats: 22.5 g
- Saturated Fat: 20.1 g
- Cholesterol: 0 mg
- Sodium: 99 mg
- Carbs: 24.8 g
- Fiber: 3.6 g
- Sugar: 14.1 g
- Protein: 2.3 g

49. Avocado Pudding

Preparation Time: 15 minutes
Cooking Time: 3 hours and 15 minutes
Servings: 4
Ingredients:

- 2 cups bananas, peeled and chopped
- 2 ripe avocados, peeled, pitted, and chopped
- 1 tsp. fresh lime zest, grated finely
- 1 tsp. fresh lemon zest, grated finely
- ½ cup fresh lime juice
- ½ cup fresh lemon juice
- ⅓ cup agave nectar

Directions:

1. In a blender, add all the ingredients and pulse until smooth.
2. Transfer the mousse into 4 serving glasses and refrigerate to chill for about 3 hours before serving.

Nutrition:

- Calories: 462
- Fats: 20.1 g
- Saturated Fat: 4.4 g
- Cholesterol: 0 mg
- Sodium: 13 mg
- Carbs: 48.2 g
- Fiber: 10.2 g
- Sugar: 30.4 g
- Protein: 3 g

50. Mini Pea Pancakes

Preparation Time: 5 minutes
Cooking Time: 15 minutes
Servings: 4
Ingredients:

- ¼ cup whole wheat flour
- ¼ cup almond flour
- 1 ½ tsp. baking powder
- 3 egg whites
- 2 cups butter milk
- 1 ¼ cup frozen peas, defrosted
- Sunflower oil spray, for frying
- ⅓ cup water

Directions:

1. Combine the flour and baking powder in a bowl.
2. Whisk the egg whites with buttermilk and ⅓ cup of water.
3. Stir in the flour mixture and mix well.
4. Fold in peas and keep the mixture aside.
5. Preheat a greased frying pan, and add flour batter spoon by spoon.
6. Cook them for 2 minutes per side.
7. Serve.

Nutrition:

- Calories: 252
- Fats: 16 g
- Saturated Fat: 7 g
- Cholesterol: 11 mg
- Sodium: 8 mg
- Carbs: 29 g
- Sugar: 1.8 g
- Fiber: 5 g
- Protein: 4 g

Conclusion

Acid Reflux Diet" is an alternative lifestyle and diet designed to help people fight back mild acid reflux by limiting or eliminating certain foods. One of the main goals of this diet is to avoid overconsumption of dairy products, which can often lead to heartburn. In addition, it promotes a low-calorie intake consisting primarily of fruit, vegetables, and lean protein sources. By eating on this particular diet plan for 3 weeks, you may be able to control your acid reflux symptoms effectively. It's not easy or simple, but it pays off in the long run!

As we end this book, here are some guidelines for you to consider when undergoing an acid reflux diet:

- Excess consumption of dairy products is one of the main culprits for causing acid reflux. You should therefore try to limit how much milk, cheese, and other dairy products you eat. If you have to eat any of these things, it's best to do so out of sight and mind, like at a restaurant instead of at home.
- Although certain foods may increase heartburn (such as spicy dishes or foods high in fat), there are also many foods you can eat that will help in combating it.
- Try not to overeat, and make sure you leave a little bit on your plate after each meal to keep your acid reflux symptoms at bay!
- Avoid eating big meals at night; try to split your daily intake of calories and nutrients among 3 smaller meals rather than 2 large ones.
- If you have any underlying heart or digestive disorders, always speak with a medical professional before starting this diet.
- If you have a past of heartburn or acid reflux, it's possible that you could end up developing ulcers (open sores) in your throat. If this occurs, then you should immediately seek the advice of your doctor.
- Understand the signs and symptoms of acid reflux as well as heartburn so that you can know if you're suffering from these conditions or have a similar illness like GERD.
- Consult your doctor about any medications or over-the-counter remedies you intend to take for heartburn and acid reflux—many medications are unsafe for use when pregnant or breastfeeding!
- Always be sure to chew your food thoroughly when eating to increase digestive efficiency and improve overall health.
- Avoid smoking or drinking large amounts of alcohol and caffeinated beverages.
- Make sure that you're taking in an adequate amount of fiber by eating many servings of fresh fruits and vegetables.
- Keep your diet very clean. Try to avoid eating anything that you wouldn't want someone to eat in front of you.
- Avoid drinking sodas, caffeinated teas, and chocolate drinks. These are all common causes of acid reflux in some people.
- Try to avoid high-fat foods, such as hamburgers, pastries, ice cream, and fatty meats (like chicken and pork).

Thank you for your time and attention.
I hope this book will help you to understand the reasons for acid reflux and, in turn, improve your health.
Good luck and good health!

Thank you for reading This book.
If you enjoyed it please visit the site where you
Purchased it and write a brief review. Your Feedback is important to me
and will help other readers decide whether to read the book too.

Thank You

Printed in Great Britain
by Amazon

78037615R00079